DEDICATION

To Majorie, Maren, and Joshua

ACKNOWLEDGMENTS

I first wish to give thanks to all the many people who work in the business of producing a book. Of special importance to me have been the editors Martha Jablow, Mary Ann Lynch, Betsy Thorpe, and Francesca Drago. I give thanks to all the people associated with Wiley.

I also wish to give thanks to those in the teaching profession, especially those teachers that not only challenge us to think more but also challenge us to do more. My favorites have been Bob Blanchard, David Till, Mary Lou Mohr, Lori Russell-Chapin, and Michael Maher.

I also wish to give thanks to all my family and friends who have offered emotional support to me during the writing of this book. I wish to especially thank my partner Mary whose gifts of love, understanding, patience, and humor have been much needed and appreciated.

Finally, I wish to give thanks to the hospice team of workers, especially the most important persons on the hospice team, the patients. Their courage, sacrifices, and mere presence provide treasures that cannot be found anywhere else.

Douglas C. Smith

CONTENTS

INTRODUCTION

For the past decade, I have worked with people who are seriously ill and dying, many of them in hospice programs around the country. I have earned two advanced degrees in hospice work, done patient care for three hospices, and taught workshops at over one hundred hospices from Florida to California to Hawaii to Minnesota to Maine and in between. While continuing to do those workshops, I am currently executive director of a hospice that has a daily patient census in excess of 100 terminally ill people. But even before all of this, death and dying were all too familiar to me: I had already lost a father, a brother, and a daughter.

My own personal experiences, my professional work experiences, and the experiences of the many people who have attended my workshops have provided me with the inspiration and information for this book.

Over the years, I have come to know scores of courageous people as well as many who are frightened, angry, lonely, or in a turmoil of conflicting emotions as the end of their lives approaches. I have listened to their questions and concerns, held their hands, prayed and meditated with them, and sat by their bedsides in silence as they slept. Each one has taught me something about the human spirit. They have given me more than I could ever have given them.

Each of these individuals had a unique story. Through this book, I will share several of their stories with those of you who now find yourselves in the position of caring for a loved one or patient who is ill, frail, or near death. You may be a relative, friend, nurse, doctor, social worker, hospice volunteer, member of the clergy, home healthcare aide—all of you are caregivers. My hope is that these stories can help all of us understand, appreciate, and promote the needs and rights of those who are approaching their last days.

Each of the stories included illustrates the basic premise of this book and of my work with hospices across the country: People who are seriously ill and dying have rights that the rest of us often overlook. They are just as entitled to these rights as all of us are to those guaranteed by the Bill of Rights in the United States Constitution. I have drafted a "Bill of Patient's Rights" that I believe are as inalienable for seriously ill and dying people as are those enacted for all Americans in 1791. You will find this "Bill of Patient's Rights" on page xvii. This book is organized around these rights, with one chapter devoted to each.

First, I offer pertinent stories drawn from my experiences and then various activites and techniques available to the caregiver. Most are for caregivers to use with the person in their care, but some are for the caregiver's benefit as well, such as activities that help reduce stress. And a few of the exercises near the end of the book are meant for families and friends to help them better understand the dying process and how to prepare for the loss of their loved ones.

In the following pages you will find a wide variety of tools and techniques for promoting patients' rights, from visualizations and then guided imagery, to meditation and "life review" techniques. All of these have been used beneficially by numerous therapists and caregivers, and I have found them all useful at different times. Not every exercise will be appropriate or comfortable for everyone: discuss them, both with the individuals in your care and with other people who are involved in their care, and select those that suit your circumstance.

The ideas behind my "Bill of Patient's Rights" were germinating at an early point in my hospice work, but they blossomed into a written document on the day after a brave, determined man I knew named Gary died. Because Gary was inspirational to me in this work, I introduce him here as a prelude to the "Bill of Patient's Rights."

Gary

Gary had been quite athletic, a marathon runner, in fact, before he was diagnosed with amyotrophic lateral sclerosis (ALS), more commonly known as Lou Gehrig's disease. ALS starts at a lower part of the body and causes progressive, upward paralysis, but the mind remains clear as ALS climbs "up the body."

Gary's paralysis began at his feet five years before I met him. When his feet first began to weaken, he felt a searing loss in his life of his role as a runner, but he was determined not to give up on maintaining a sense of purpose. He continued going to work although he had to use a wheelchair. As the paralysis progressed, Gary needed to ask for assistance with simple things, like reaching books that were on a high shelf. He became increasingly dependent on employees who had long been dependent on him, to the humiliating point of once having to ask for help in getting off a toilet.

Although Gary finally had to quit his job, he still refused to give up hope. While he could no longer run and work at his old job, he decided he could still work at something. He started a local support group for people with ALS and their families, and began to give talks throughout the community. I met Gary when he gave a presentation to a hospice volunteer training program with which I was involved.

At first Gary traveled to his speaking engagements in a specially equipped van that he could drive himself. But with the ever-enchroaching paralysis, he was soon unable to drive the van. Once more, Gary would not surrender his sense of purpose. By this time he had only partial use of one arm so he added a unique swivel device to his computer that permitted him to operate it with his good hand floating freely above the keyboard. Working with his computer and modem, Gary was able to play a key role in researching and designing hardware and software for the network of computers used by the hospice that was assisting him with his care.

Eventually, ALS's progressive paralysis stole Gary's ability to operate the computer. But before that loss, he had entered into his computer a eulogy and all other funeral arrangements that he wanted, including the names and telephone numbers of everyone he wished to be contacted upon his death. With every bit of strength he had left and every shred of willpower he could muster, Gary did what he could to stay active and maintain a sense of purpose. He exercised as much control as he could over his destiny until the very end.

The day after Gary died, many of the ideas and experiences I had shared with him and others crystallized into a "Bill of Patient's Rights." I hope that you will read it, think seriously about it, share it with those in your care, and perhaps put it near their bedside for others to consider. By working together with other caregivers, relatives, and friends—and with our loved ones and patients who are able to participate—we can collectively improve their lives with the gifts of dignity and respect. We can turn these rights into opportunities that will enrich the quality each day. As we interact on a daily basis, we can keep our twofold task in the forefront of our minds: to keep them alive and simultaneously help them learn how to die.

A BILL OF PATIENT'S RIGHTS

The Right to Be in Control

Grant me the right to make as many decisions as possible regarding my care. Please do not take choices from me. Let me make my own decisions.

The Right to Have a Sense of Purpose

I have lost my job. I can no longer fulfill my role in my family. Please help me find some new sense of purpose.

The Right to Reminisce

There has been pleasure in my life, moments of pride, moments of love. Please give me some time to recollect those moments. And please listen to my recollections.

The Right to Know the Truth

When you withhold the truth from me, you treat me as if I am no longer living. I am still living, and I need to know the truth about my life. Please help me find that truth.

The Right to Be in Denial

If I hear the truth and choose not to accept it, that is my right.

The Right to Be Comfortable

The pain involved in dying is multifaceted. Although not all my pain can be taken away, please relieve whatever portion you can.

continued

The Right to Touch and Be Touched

Sometimes I need distance. Yet sometimes I have a strong need to be close. When I want to reach out, please come to me and hold me as I hold you.

The Right to Laughter

People often—far too often—come to me wearing masks of seriousness. Although dying, I still need to laugh. Please laugh with me and help others to laugh as well.

The Right to Cry and Express Anger

It is difficult to leave behind all my attachments and all that I love. Please allow me the opportunity to be sad and angry.

The Right to Explore the Spiritual

Whether I am questioning or affirming, doubting or praising, I sometimes need your ear, a nonjudgmental ear. Please let my spirit travel its own journey, without judging its direction.

The Right to Have a Sense of Family

No matter what defines my present family—it may be a small circle of friends and caregivers; it may encompass relatives or not—I have need, now more than ever, to experience the connectedness, the intimacy, and the interdependence that constitute family.

Please honor all my rights. One day, you too will want these same rights.

CHAPTER ONE

The Right to Be in Control

The process of dying can be devastating. It can be brief or prolonged. It can be ugly and often heart-wrenching. But it can also provide moments that are profoundly enriching, both for the person nearing the end of life and for family members and caregivers. What makes the difference? What factors can enrich those last months or hours?

The answer lies in the attitudes and practices of the caregiver, whether that person is a relative, friend, volunteer, or professional. The people surrounding a seriously ill or dying person can make all the difference. They can promote and ensure a patient's rights to a sense of purpose, control, comfort, laughter, touch, reminiscence, spirituality, truth or denial—the rights that enrich the process of dying—or they can rob patients of those rights and diminish their final days.

No caregiver would consciously or deliberately try to diminish a person's life during its final phases, but we often do so unintentionally: "Here, eat just another spoonful of applesauce . . . Now, take your pill, dear; you know it will make you feel better . . . Oh, here, I'll do that for you . . ." We can sound as though we are talking to a two-year-old instead of an adult, an adult who has lived a full and independent life. We assume that because we are stronger, more able-bodied, and perhaps even better informed, we naturally know what is best.

But we need to be aware that people in the final phases of their lives lose many choices and freedoms from big choices, like deciding upon a course of medical treatment, to smaller, formerly routine choices like what clothes to wear today or what to eat for lunch. Forms of control are stolen from them continually, eroded away by external forces. They lose many abilities and opportunities that younger or healthier people take for granted: a simple walk outside; the option of social-izing with whomever they choose (rather than the chatterbox in the next bed or the dour fellow who always eats at their table in the nursing home's dining room); the capacity to eliminate various aches and pains; sometimes even the loss of bodily functions.

These losses are often coupled with the loss of major roles that previously identified and made up their lives—a job, a place in society, and participation in the community. They may no longer be able to volunteer for a neighborhood event or fill a long-standing position in their religious organiza-tion. Hobbies and pastimes may become sharply curtailed: they cannot bend to tee up a golf ball, swing a tennis racquet, or get down on their hands and knees to pull weeds from the garden. And at the same time, their family role may become greatly diminished. A once strong, decisive parent may have to yield duties and prerogatives—maintaining the home, pay-ing the bills, making financial decisions—to someone else.

With such significant losses, people with drastically impaired functions or in the final phases of life hunger for any kind of control they can grasp in their day-to-day lives. The tighter the rein their illness has on them, the more they want to keep it at bay by maintaining some sort of control, any type of control. No one, of course, ever has complete control over life, but each of us has a right to be in some control regardless of our age or health status. Those in the later stages of life do not and should not relinquish that right with their illness and may, in fact, desire some measure of control precisely because so much else has been lost.

The right to be in control throughout one's life is a basic human right. The extent to which each individual can exercise that right is determined by their own physical and mental condition, but that right should be guaranteed and nurtured as much as possible by the rest of us.

To underscore this right, I want to relate the stories of four people whose lives illustrate the importance of the right to be in control. At first, you may not agree with the paths that each took near the end of their lives. You may be uncomfortable with or not approve of their denial, anger, noncompliance with a medical regimen, or with the refusal to let go of life in the face of overwhelming odds. But if you listen to these stories with an open heart and mind, you may understand why I have chosen to introduce you to these people who exemplify the right to be in control.

Martha

Cancer had metastasized throughout Martha's 80-year-old body. Her condition was apparent to her family, friends, and medical advisors, but Martha refused to allow the word "cancer" to be spoken in her presence. In discussing her illness, she used the phrase "the naughty word." She also refused to let anyone around her mention the words "dying" or "death." Whenever any of those words were inadvertently mentioned, she turned away from the speaker, faced the nearest wall, and thrashed her arms in agitation.

Although many people may think Martha's attitude was unrealistic or childish, it was her right to request that certain words not be spoken in her presence. This was the way she chose to control her environment at the end of her life. Her principal caregiver decided to honor Martha's particular method of control because she recognized Martha's right to exercise some degree of control, to set her own agenda, to be free of the labels of others. This was her right and her style of exercising that right.

A dying person needs to be shown unconditional love, free of our expectations and judgments. Another caregiver might have tried to "reason" with Martha to persuade her to accept her cancer, her coming death, and the spoken use of their names. But that would have been an imposition of the caregiver's opinions.

The physical and mental deterioration that usually accompanies the dying process is experienced as an imposition by the patient. Outside factors are knocking at the door, pushing their way in uninvited, stealing health, happiness, and control. So much had intruded on Martha already that any added encumbrance from the caregiver would not have been welcome.

For many dying people, it can be too much to bear to have to tolerate further impositions of other peoples' theories and expectations about how to act. If Martha chose to be "irrational" by denying the words "cancer" and "death," so be it. That was her choice and her right. Certainly, she was trying to cope by using some strong denial. Yet who among us won't experience some degree of denial near the end of our lives? Some of us may end up in total denial. Should we not have that right? Should we not have the right to cope and be in control as much as we are able when we see our lives dissolving before us? People who are seriously ill, aging, or dying want and need a respectful acceptance. We will want the same someday.

Acceptance means that we caregivers impose no reservations, no conditions, no evaluations, and no judgments about our care recipient's feelings. Instead, acceptance requires that we show a total, positive regard for them as people of value, whether we agree with their attitudes, feelings, and decisions or not. This is respectful acceptance—it directs us as caregivers to become involved with a sick or dying person without imposing our own labels and expectations, even when we believe that our expectations are right, good, healthy, appropriate, or proper.

We need to be careful of the many subtle ways that we impose our beliefs on others. A self-described "recovering psychotherapist," Anne Wilson Schaef, recognized how often and how easily we indirectly or unintentionally manipulate patients:

> I began to see that thinking I knew what a person needed, or even where they were or what was

going on with them, was disrespectful and a form of control. I began to see that my subtle forms of "interpretation" were disrespectful and doing the [person's] work for him or her, which in itself is a form of disrespect. I was catching on to the myriad subtle little ways that I threw in "suggestions," "interpretations," "I remember whens," "I wonder ifs," and so on. More disrespect![1]

We caregivers need to have a respectful acceptance that allows people to retain control over their own lives.

Phyllis

Phyllis was 64 years of age, living in a nursing home, and one of the younger residents there. To those around her, Phyllis seemed determined to use her remaining energy to complain and to verbally assault anyone who came into her presence. She was not only extremely angry about the fact that her poor health necessitated her being in a nursing home, but she was also intent upon letting everyone know it. She yelled. She screamed. She attacked and accused others of every possible incursion.

This was Phyllis's choice, her method of coping, her way of expressing anger. This was how she expressed her distress at having to leave her home and family and be "confined," as she charged, to a nursing home. Expressing anger was her way of seizing some control, the only control she felt she had. Phyllis could not choose to be healthy, but she could choose to be angry about being unhealthy. She could not choose to live where she wished, but she could choose to be angry about where she felt she was "forced" to live. By letting everyone know of her anger, Phyllis exercised the only control she felt she had left.

One of her caregivers decided to honor Phyllis's choices by caring for her without trying to change her attitude or erase her anger. The caregiver concluded that, if Phyllis wanted to have someone to assault verbally, the caregiver would volunteer to be the target. By letting Phyllis yell, scream, insult, attack, and accuse, her caregiver honored Phyllis's choice. Her caregiver thus gave Phyllis the gift of retaining some sense of control in her life.

Phyllis's story may seem extreme to some. Why should a caregiver have to take that kind of abuse, even from a dying person? they may ask. Some professional caregivers or even loving relatives might find it easier just to distance themselves from this kind of verbal abuse. They might prefer to walk out of Phyllis's room than to take her assaults. But we must try to see the patient's point of view. Try to understand that this kind of behavior or reaction to ever-encroaching physical limitations can make some people like Phyllis grasp at any means of control, even the loudest, strongest expression of anger. Try to accept therefore, that you are not a personal target of her anger, but that her anger is aimed at her loss of control in her life.

When we hear an insult or listen to a string of angry verbal attacks, we need to try and reconsider them as a part of the ongoing care of someone whose control is being continually eroded. If we caregivers can put it in that perspective, and take ourselves figuratively out of the bull's-eye and off the target, we will not intrude. We will stop trying to take away or limit the patient's sense of control. We will not force our needs and insights on her. Thus, we can gently allow the person to exist without constricting their freedom or forcing them to act as we desire.

Charlie

At age 70, Charlie was struggling with lung cancer and chronic obstructive pulmonary disease. In his youth, he had helped his father raise tobacco. He began smoking at an early age and learned to make moonshine in the hills of Kentucky. By age 15, Charlie decided to hit the road for "the big shoulders" of Chicago. He worked as a cook, bus driver, and self-ordained minister over the years.

In his treatment regimen for lung cancer, Charlie had been receiving Dilaudid™ tablets and duragesic patches for pain. He often pretended to swallow the tablets, and he secretly took off the patches. When discovered, he said he preferred to follow his own regimen of pain control—smoking heavily, praying often, and strongly believing in a reunion with his beloved wife in heaven.

Although there was no question that pain medication brought him some comfort, Charlie liked being able to choose his own form of care. If he'd been allowed complete control, he said, he would toss out all the prescribed medications "as quick as I used to hide the moonshine from the revenuers" in the Kentucky hills.

Charlie had led a good, full life. He had exercised much independence. Should other people engage in taking some of that independence from him? Should caregivers be in the business of treating him as if he were not an adult with the same rights as the rest of us? Should we try to control him rather than allow him his own control?

Cathy

Cathy was very young to face death. At age 35, she desperately wanted to live for her young children. But everyone around her, including her parents, saw futility in her desire to live as terminal illness numbered her days. During the last week of her life, Cathy's parents were at her bedside, witnessing her pain and praying for its relief. They ardently believed that her pain could only be relieved through death so they verbally gave Cathy permission to die. They hoped that their permission could assist her in the dying process.

Cathy's parents—with completely good intentions—continued this approach for several days. As they gently rubbed her back or held her hand or stroked her hair, they told Cathy that she had fought a great, brave fight, but that it was time to let go.

Cathy's response was a resounding "No!" Despite her physical weakness, she said "No!" angrily whenever they made the suggestion or talked about "going toward the light." Her parents used guided imagery by portraying the image of a reunion with her favorite relative, her grandfather. They sometimes talked about all the good arrangements that were being made for the future care of Cathy's children. But even in a semiconscious state, Cathy always protested, "No!"

On the last day of her life, Cathy's struggle was obvious to everyone who entered her room. Some relatives, friends, and staff saw it as a conflict between the known and the unknown. Others likened it to the labor of giving birth. Some saw it as a battle with God. However interpreted, Cathy's fight was communicated through her body's writhing in physical contortions that no medication could alleviate. Throughout her final hours, she uttered the insistent "No!" It was her final word.

No one knew for certain why Cathy persisted in refusing death until it overtook her. Yet, if we are advocates for choice and control, we really don't need to know her reasons—because it was Cathy's death and no one else's. It was her resistance, her choice, that needed to be honored whether her reasons were known or unknown, accepted and agreed with or not.

———

You have just met four people who took control of their final days in different ways. Martha chose denial. Phyllis raged with anger. Charlie preferred noncompliance. And Cathy refused to let go against everyone's urging. In the traditional modes of therapy, many professionals, as well as family members, would try to eliminate that denial, suppress that anger, enforce compliance, and even railroad people into acceptance of the expectations of others.

But if we do eliminate, suppress, enforce, and railroad, we are robbing these individuals of their own control. We are exercising *our* control over people who have had to give up immense amounts of autonomy already. We are stealing their opportunity—perhaps their only and last opportunity—to have control of their own being. They are already powerless enough; we need not take away any more. The best thing we can do in assisting them during their last years and days is to promote their right to be in as much control of their lives as possible.

But how can we do that when their physical, and perhaps mental and spiritual, strength and energy are failing? The following sections offer various activities and techniques caregivers may employ to enhance their prolonged illness or patient's or loved one's sense of control.

Tools and techniques for promoting the right to be in control

ASSESSING STRENGTHS

When people who are suddenly disabled or near the end of life must enter a caregiving environment, whether in their own home, a relative's home, nursing home, or hospital, they are often subjected to something called an *assessment*. It is usually defined as a process that determines which problems are most prominent; it may be formal or informal and may be completed by relatives or professionals. From this assessment, a plan of care is developed to address and alleviate those problems.

To most family members and caregivers, it seems like an innocent, even helpful process. But think about it for a moment: Who's doing the assessment? Who is in the driver's seat? Who is in control? The usual assessment process communicates to ill or dying people that they are in need of some problem-solving, and that the assessor—not the person whose problems are being assessed—is the one who is going to solve the problems. The none-too-subtle inherent message is: Hand over control of your life to the assessor; you are no longer in control, but your caregiver/assessor is.

This approach is out of balance because it identifies one party as weak and the other as strong, one in control, the other to be controlled. This can potentially create more problems. In many instances, I have found, this problem-centered assessment can even accentuate one of the more serious situations among people in the final phases of life—the depression and despair that come from a sense of helplessness.

However, there is a way to turn this around: If caregivers assess for strengths rather than weaknesses or problems, the person being assessed will receive a positive, empowering message: "You are not out of control or losing control. You have the wherewithal to solve your own problems. You do have some control." In this way, the caregiver takes the role of a facilitator and a helper, and not some sort of psychosocial savior.

This positive type of assessment also can produce much more useful information. By the time the need for an assessment arises, the individual usually has come to require a caregiver's help with many complex, ever-changing, medical and psychological problems. When the traditional, problem-centered type of assessment is done, the focus is narrow: What is the problem currently? But these needs and problems change, sometimes daily.

If, on the other hand, a strength-centered assessment is done, caregivers gain a broader perspective. Caregiver and patient together can consider qualities that have developed over time, perhaps over a lifetime. In widening their focus and looking for strengths, caregivers can discover vital information that is of lasting value over the course of the illness or dying process. For example, a person may have a longtime love of music that can be put to good use in relaxation or meditation efforts during periods of physical discomfort. Another patient may rely on a personal faith for coping— a strength that can again be called upon during the current illness.

A person's problems continually change in category, type, and degree of severity, but established strengths can be reinforced from day to day once the caregiver is aware of them. In assessing for strengths, caregiver and patient can investigate a coping style used over a lifetime of "little deaths," a coping style that has resulted in survival and growth and that can now be called upon as reinforcement to face today's issues. Those little deaths might include the first day we entered a new school, the time a close friend moved away, the day we left home to work on our own, the first time our children went to school, the day we lost a job or got a divorce, the time a loved one died, or many other occasions of loss. The coping strengths that were developed in each case can help with adjustment to the current situation.

In the following assessment procedure, the emphasis is on strengths because this approach can communicate a sense of control to the sick or dying person. By focusing on strengths rather than problems, caregivers can assist patients to uncover their own resources, resources that can help alleviate stress, offer more choices, and allow increased control over daily life. Of the five questions that follow, you may decide to ask all five, only two or three, or just the first question. The point is simply to turn the spotlight away from problems and onto strengths that increase the patient's right to be in control.

A Strength Assessment

1. What are your three greatest strengths?
2. How would you summarize, in one or two sentences, your philosophy for getting through the rough times and getting enjoyment out of life?

3. When family and friends have turned to you for help, what kind of help have they been seeking?

4. When your life is over, what things are people going to miss most about you?

5. When the time comes for someone to write your eulogy, what contributions are they going to say that you gave to your community? your family?

The next task for the caregiver is to use productively the information gathered from this assessment. For example, if you have discovered that one of the greatest strengths of your patient is faith, you can remind her to draw on that when conditions grow difficult. If another patient's greatest strength is humor, you can tap into that when he is going through a period of low self-worth. Such information is valuable no matter what the person's current problems are, no matter how complex they may become. Perhaps the most valuable benefit of assessing strengths is the control it allows the patient to retain. When we discover strengths and remind our patient of them, we enable the patient to enjoy a sense of self-worth, to exercise self-help, and, especially, to feel a sense of control.

Certainly, there is a need to investigate problems as well, and this strength assessment exercise is not intended to downplay that requirement. But too often strengths are overshadowed by problems, so we need to put a little more effort into looking for strengths that can buoy a patient's sense of control.

Conversations that Nourish

In the same positive spirit as emphasizing strengths, professional and nonprofessional caregivers need to choose their words carefully in everyday conversations with those in their care. Instead of the daily question, "What problems are you having today?" we can occasionally ask, "What successes have you felt today?"

Instead of always posing the question, "Where do you hurt?" or "Where is the pain?" we could occasionally inquire, "Where do you feel good?" And in place of the usual, "Can I help you?" we need to ask once in a while, "Am I being too helpful?"

When we continually remind people of the bad things in their lives, rather than the good, we are telling them that they do not have enough strength to help themselves. When we constantly offer to help them without allowing them to help themselves, we are actually stealing positive energy from them. And of course, word by word, we are eroding their sense of control.

But if we direct the conversation toward the good aspects of their lives rather than dwelling on the negatives, we can allow people to be in touch with their positive energy, and we can therefore help fuel that energy. By promoting and participating in such nourishing conversations, we are enabling them to have a sense of control.

ALLOWING YOUR ROLE TO BE DEFINED

As we have just recognized, the typical assessment process tends to give control to the assessor rather than to the person who is being assessed. But it is possible to give even more control to recipients of our care, instead of taking it from them. The following assessment forms are intended to help you in your specific caregiving role, as well as the person in your care, achieve several goals. These forms, directed to both patient and caregiver needs, can produce uniquely beneficial results:

- The forms allow care receivers some choice in defining various caregivers' roles. This helps to clarify each caregiver's relationship, responsibility, and function. Such clarification may seem obvious to some, but it is important because many people with restricted abilities or in the final phases of life are confused about what roles their cast of caregivers will play. For example, what is the doctor's precise role, and how does it differ from the social worker's? Who is expected to make certain arrangements for care? How does the home healthcare aide's role differ from the visiting nurse's? What is a family member's role and responsibility in the broader scope of overall care?

- The forms allow care receivers some choice in setting priorities in your mutual relationship. This lets them know from the outset that they control the relationship rather than the other way around. These forms also offer care receivers the ability to define boundaries and off-limit topics. This is significant because it prevents caregivers from inadvertently raising an issue or performing a procedure that the recipient does not want.

Xerox these assessment forms so they can be easily used by your care recipient. As you offer them, keep in mind that you are switching roles with the people who receive your care. You are giving them greater control than they have previously had. Ideally, these forms should be shared with them at the outset, when you first enter their environment. But if you are already in an ongoing relationship, it is not too late to initiate these forms. You will find that they have a dual benefit: They not only give care receivers more control, but they also let caregivers know exactly what is expected of them.

Ask your patients if they would prefer to fill out the forms alone or if they would like you to be with them. Often, patients will prefer doing this activity on their own time and at their own pace. Ask them, in this case, when it would be convenient for you to retrieve the forms; and when you do, be sure to talk with them about the forms before you even begin to look at them. You may find that the simple act of letting them state what they want and do not want will open a new level of dialogue, intimacy, and trust.

Social Worker or Counselor Role Definition

From the following list of items that you, the care recipient, might receive from your caregiver, put an "x" beside those that best complete this statement: "I would like my social worker or counselor to help me. . . ." Cross out any item that you feel you will never want from a caregiver. Put a question mark next to any you are unsure about. Use the blank space for anything else you wish to say.

I would like my social worker or counselor to help me. . .

_____ learn more about my illness/condition;

_____ explore nonmedical ways of relieving pain or anxiety;

_____ learn how to give and receive touching better;

_____ put some fun and humor into my life;

_____ explore religious or spiritual issues;

_____ address money issues (medical costs, wills, etc.);

_____ make more decisions about my own well-being;

_____ accept my restricted life conditions;

_____ accept my limited life span;

_____ explore nursing homes or other living arrangements;

_____ communicate feelings toward a particular person (_____);

_____ finish a project (_____);

_____ something else (_____).

Nursing Role Definition

From the following list of items that you, the care recipient, would like to receive from your nurse, put an "x" beside those that best complete this statement: "I would like my nurse to help me. . . ." Cross out any item that you feel you will never want from a nurse. Put a question mark next to any you are unsure about. Use the blank space for anything else you wish to say.

I would like my nurse to help me. . .

_____ find medication for pain relief;

_____ find medication for other physical problems;

_____ address some emotional issues;

_____ learn more about alternatives to pain
        medication;

_____ learn about ways to put more quality into
        my life;

_____ understand the length and status of my last
        days;

_____ communicate with my physician(s);

_____ make more decisions about my own
        well-being;

_____ adjust to loss of control over bodily
        functions;

_____ communicate my concerns and wishes to
        my family and close friends;

_____ explore religious or spiritual issues;

_____ communicate feelings toward a particular
        person (_____);

_____ finish a project (_____);

_____something else (_____).

Chaplain Role Definition

From the following list of items that you, the care recipient, might receive from your chaplain, put an "x" beside those that best complete this statement: "I would like my chaplain to help me. . . ." Cross out any item that you feel you will never want from a chaplain. Put a question mark next to any you are unsure about. Use the blank space for anything else you wish to say.

I would like my chaplain to help me. . .

_____ maintain contact with my congregation, minister, rabbi, or priest;

_____ strengthen my life with prayer and/or meditation;

_____ explore some of my spiritual concerns;

_____ feel a sense of worth and dignity;

_____ settle some religious differences within my family;

_____ look at planning for my funeral service;

_____ talk about an afterlife;

_____ help a particular member of my family;

_____ find some good reading or study materials for my struggles;

_____ address some of my doubts, fears, and/or anger;

_____ find a clergyperson and/or congregation;

_____ something else (_____).

Home Health Aide Role Definition

From the following list of items that you, the care recipient, might receive from your home health aide, put an "x" beside those that best complete this statement: "I would like my home health aide to help me. . . ." Cross out any item that you feel you will never want from a home health aide. Put a question mark next to any you are unsure about. Use the blank space for anything else you wish to say.

I would like my home health aide to help me . . .

_____ bathe and clean myself;

_____ dress myself;

_____ take care of grooming matters;

_____ maintain a clean and safe environment;

_____ retrain for necessary self-help skills;

_____ use and exercise my muscle groups;

_____ achieve more mobility;

_____ massage away soreness and tension;

_____ purchase, prepare, and/or serve meals;

_____ do light housekeeping;

_____ finish a project (_____);

_____ something else (_____).

Volunteer Role Definition

From the following list of items that you, the care recipient, might receive from your volunteer, put an "x" beside those that best complete this statement: "I would like my volunteer to help me. . . ." Cross out any item that you feel you will never want from a volunteer. Put a question mark next to any you are unsure about. Use the blank space for anything else you wish to say.

I would like my volunteer to. . .

_____ give me some occasional companionship;

_____ relieve some of my other caregivers of their duties;

_____ put some fun and humor into my life;

_____ read to me and/or write for me;

_____ help me with housekeeping matters;

_____ help me plan for my family's future;

_____ run some errands outside the home;

_____ help me do some "handyman" projects;

_____ explore religious/spiritual issues;

_____ finish a project (_____);

_____ do something else (_____).

Family Member Role Definition

From the following list of items that you, the care recipient, might receive from your family member, put an "x" beside those that best complete this statement: "I would like my family member to help me. . . ." Cross out any item that you feel you will never want from a family member. Put a question mark next to any you are unsure about. Use the blank space for anything else you wish to say.

I would like my family member to help me. . .

_____ review my life;

_____ plan for my family's future;

_____ address money issues (medical costs, wills, etc.);

_____ feel a sense of worth and dignity;

_____ express touch through holding and hugging;

_____ talk about some emotional issues;

_____ put some fun and humor into my life;

_____ explore religious/spiritual issues;

_____ communicate with someone
(_____);

_____ finish a project (_____);

_____ do something else (_____).

DIALOGUE WITH DEATH

Much of the stress felt by people in their final years comes from the natural sense of having no control over death. We feel death is an inevitable reality we cannot avoid, that it will arrive in its own time and that we cannot schedule it—either postpone or hurry its arrival.

Yet we can have some control over death itself. In hospice work, we see this control proven by statistics that show how often people die shortly after a holiday, right after an anniversary, or soon after a specific person's visit rather than before each of these significant events. We frequently see dying patients consciously fend off death until they feel they have reached an appropriate time or until a certain milestone is attained. This demonstrates that they do indeed have some control over the timing of their own deaths. The dying often go through a period of resisting death before moving into another phase of welcoming it.

Dying patients may be unaware of the control they possess. Caregivers can help them to become more keenly aware of their control, and can help alleviate their patients' and loved ones' natural fear of having no influence over the arrival and timing of their own death. One useful technique that caregivers can use to promote this awareness is the following "Dialogue with Death." This is an imagery experience; that is, an experience that requires the dying person to imagine talking face-to-face with a figure personifying death itself. Some readers may think that this is too much to ask of a dying person, one who is perhaps frail, elderly, anxious, or depressed. But we have found that many people in the final phases of life have already been conversing with death, and their dialogues have been quite frightening. This guided imagery exercise can help to ease their fears.

I would suggest that, as caregiver, you read the imagery dialogue with pauses between sentences to allow your care recipients an opportunity to verbalize the images, thoughts, and responses that come to mind. Or you may want to suggest that they listen silently and later write or dictate a report of the images and responses that they imagined as you read the dialogue aloud. You can ask the person you are caring for which option is preferable. Before beginning this dialogue, I would also suggest that you may want to adapt the same format for different occasions; it could also be reworded as a "Dialogue with Pain" or a "Dialogue with Stress."

DIALOGUE WITH DEATH

Close your eyes and imagine yourself sitting across from an empty chair. Now imagine that the personification of death is sitting in that chair. What would Death look like if it were a person sitting there? . . . What does the face of Death look like? . . . Describe the clothes that Death is wearing. . . . What do the hands of Death look like?

What would you want to say to Death? . . . Verbalize what you want to say in the present tense, just as though Death is actually sitting in that chair across from you. . . . Say everything you want to say to Death.

Now put yourself in that chair and visualize yourself as Death looking at you. Verbalize Death's response to you. If you were Death, what would you say to the person in front of you? Say everything that Death would say. . . . How would Death respond to the message that you had previously directed toward Death?

Although you cannot eliminate the existence of Death, you have the power to exercise some control over Death. In replying to what Death has just said, go back in your imagination to your original place and tell Death what you want Death to do. Verbalize some orders to Death. Tell Death how you expect Death to behave from this moment forward. . . . Tell Death also how you want Death to change in physical appearance, and say what you expect Death to wear for the next visit.

Now tell Death to get up from the chair and leave the room. . . . As you visualize Death starting to exit, tell Death that you realize that you will see Death again, but you expect Death to wait for an invitation before coming to see you again.

For the present moment, say good-bye to Death . . . and slowly open your eyes. . . .

People in the midst of the dying process often come to know when it is a good moment to welcome death. They often arrive at a place where they want death to come to them. This verbal imaging exercise can demonstrate how much control people have over death by allowing the patient to actually order death around. As the patient participates in this, she exercises considerable power in determining not only what death looks like, but even what death does and says. This experience can leave the patient with realistic hope that she indeed has some sense of control over how, and even when, her death will arrive.

WHAT A WAY TO GO: A PLAN FOR DEATH

In this activity, a caregiver can suggest a blueprint for the best, or most appropriate, way to die. You may begin by reading the following:

> There is an assignment that I invite you to do. I would like you to write what I call a "healthy death" story over the next few days. In your story, imagine the best possible death that can happen to you. Your story should have only elements that are actually possible: your best possible death.
>
> Mention how you die, what you look like, who is with you, what your thoughts are, and what you are doing as you die. Go into a lot of detail, and let your imagination run freely as you imagine an ideal death that is also a possible death.
>
> The next time we are together, we can review your story. If you prefer to draw a picture of your death rather than write a story, go ahead. We can

discuss that when we next visit. Then, each time we meet in the future, we can explore ways that might make part of your story come closer to reality.

Whether we are professional or nonprofessional caregivers, we can be architects helping the people in our care to design their own individual plans for an ideal death. We can use this picture as a blueprint for their caregiving.

This exercise may also be modified to address other areas, such as "A Plan for an Ideal Family Visit" or "A Plan for a Perfect Weekend." In many institutions, typical plans of care are multipage documents listing all potential problems and ways to address them. Those care plans rarely mention anything about a dying person's wishes, hopes, and dreams. The ideal plan described through the exercise above can be a very helpful substitute for, or accompaniment to, those traditional plans of care. If we truly want to care for people, doesn't it make far more sense to address their wishes, hopes, ideals, and dreams as well as their problems?

In reality, it may not be possible to fulfill all of their wishes literally, but that does not mean that we caregivers cannot try to create some semblance of those wishes. For instance, those distant, long-lost relatives might be unable to fly across the country for one last visit, but a caregiver might be able to arrange a phone call or suggest that they make a video- or audiotape to send to the dying patient.

If a dying person's story includes an unachievable dream to die under a palm tree on a sandy beach in Hawaii, a caregiver could creatively transform a little of that dream into reality by bringing in a lei, a large picture of the beach, a pineapple milkshake, some recordings of Hawaiian music, or tapes of breaking ocean waves. Although this is a small piece of the dying person's ideal death scenario, it can help to give some sense of control in the overall plan of care.

FROM "I NEED" TO "I CAN GET"

The following activity can enhance patients' sense of control by adapting a technique from the "rational emotive therapy" school of psychology, a form of therapy that emphasizes self-empowerment. In this exercise, care recipients are led to the realization that they have choices they may not know they have, choices they can exercise if they wish. The activity has three steps led by a caregiver with input from the patient:

1. The caregiver would assign "homework" to complete twelve sentences that each begin with the phrase "I need. . . ." The care receiver might complete the sentences, for example, "I need people to touch and hold me." Or, "I need some private time."

2. From the list of twelve needs, the caregiver may select three to five that could become your caregiving goals. In each of those three to five statements, you would replace "I need . . ." with "I can get. . . ." ("I can get people to touch and hold me." "I can get some private time.")

3. After choosing the "I can get" statements, you would write each statement on a separate sheet of paper and help your patient or loved one determine a strategy for making that statement a reality. Several different strategies may be incorporated to accomplish the goals defined in the "I can get" statements. You might

decide, for example, to set aside fifteen minutes each afternoon for your patient to be alone for that desired "private time." You could put a PLEASE DO NOT DISTURB UNTIL 4:30 sign on the door to prevent interruptions. You could also explain to the others who come in contact with your patient or loved one that she wants this private time, and ask them to respect it.

With this exercise, patients can have the satisfaction of gaining immediate results they have brought about by naming their goals.

AFFIRMATIONS

The use of "affirmations" is a technique that for years has been found helpful to change and improve a person's mental and physical health. Affirmations are easily adaptable for people in their final years. The technique works like this: You, the caregiver, ask your care recipient to choose one to three affirmations that are the most appealing from the following list. Write these down and have your care recipient verbalize these affirmations several times each day. These written statements could be placed throughout the living space as handy reminders.

If you are a family member or friend initiating this activity, you may want to tell the professional caregivers about it. Or if you are the social worker, nurse, or other professional, you may want to share the results of this activity with the family and friends. The wider the circle of caregivers who are aware of the patient's affirmations, the better. When times become difficult, you can remind the person in your care of his or her affirmations. By going back and reviewing these affirmations, you help your patient continue the quest for experiences that give a sense of control, self-help, and self-worth.

The following fourteen affirmations are simply suggestions. The person in your care may want to create his or her own affirmation statements. (One woman in a Boston intensive care unit, for example, created her own unique statement: "I will feel 36 percent better tomorrow!")

1. Every day, in every way, I am getting more at peace with myself, my family, my environment.

2. I am a powerful person because I am filled with love.

3. I accept and love myself just as I am.

4. The more I love myself, the more I can love others.

5. I have already done what I have needed to do with my life.

6. My life has truly been full of joy.

7. It is my right to enjoy my life, and I do.

8. I am a temple in which the spirit of God dwells.

9. This is a day that God has made, and I rejoice to see it.

10. I am letting go of my life in peace and joy.

11. I will make every day of my life a day in which I will learn something new.

12. Everyday I will make at least one person smile.

13. My body might be leaving this world, but my influence will remain.

14. I will be fondly remembered for many things.

Many books and calendars are also available in bookstores and libraries, full of daily affirmations that may help to offer a fresh perspective every day.

CONTROLLING PAIN AND STRESS

We all have the power to control the intensity of our pain and stress, to some extent, through our imaginations. The following imagery experience attempts to bring this control to people in our care. The experience can be verbalized by you, memorized by the person in your care, or tape-recorded in your voice or his. It is most useful to record it, of course, because the tape can be replayed whenever pain or stress arises.

A WALK ON THE OCEAN BEACH

Without a care in the world, you are walking along a beach. You are breathing the fresh ocean air. . . . You feel the summer air fill your lungs with gentle warmth. You feel the air's warmth swirl into, and throughout, your lungs. . . . It is about five o'clock in the afternoon and the sun is just resting above the horizon, about to go to sleep for the night. The sun is a brilliant, glowing orange. The sky is a hazy blue. The sand beneath your feet is a warm, soothing beige. . . . You can feel the massaging warmth of the sand through your toes as you walk. . . .

Your lips are brushed with a thin coating of salt. You lick your lips and taste the salt. . . . You hear the refreshing splashes of the waves coming in and going out,

continued

---

coming in and going out with the same rhythm as your breathing, the breathing of the fresh ocean air. . . . A distant seagull, flying toward the setting sun, cries out. Its cries become more and more distant. . . .

As you are walking, you see in front of you a sand dune, bending and bulging on the horizon. The dune is covered with flowers, splashes of yellow, blue, orange, pink. . . . You reach the sand dune and sit down, stretch your arms to the sky, and gaze in wonder out to the sea. The ocean shimmers in silver, reflecting the last rays of the setting sun. . . . As the sun slowly dips into the water, you become more and more relaxed. The lower the sun, the deeper your relaxation. . . . The warmth of the ocean air enters your lungs and relaxes you even more, and more. . . . All of your being begins to be absorbed into everything that surrounds you. You are the radiant sun. You are the shimmering sea. You are the massaging warmth of the sand. You are the flowers splashed with color. You are the ocean air swirling in your lungs. You are the distant gull crying in joy to the horizon. You are the world at peace, at rest, comfortable, relaxed. . . .

This particular example of guided imagery capitalizes on a sick or dying person's own powers of sight, sound, smell, and touch. As in other similar exercises, care receivers are guided to an awareness of their own strengths, rather than relying on some external source of strength. Once again, we are trying to help them become active rather than passive participants in their own care by centering on their right to be in control.

Care receivers can exercise even more control if we care-givers get material for guided imagery exercises from them directly. For example, during a time when they are relatively relaxed and out of pain, ask them to tell you about a time in the past when they were very comfortable. Select details from the patient's own remembrance and use them to fashion a new guided imagery activity appropriate to the individual person.

If the patient tells you, for instance, that she remembers a particularly relaxing time at a mountain cabin with her spouse, a weekend getaway soon after their last child left home, you could create this guided imagery:

> Close your eyes. . . . Remember the time you de-scribed to me, the weekend when you went to the moun-tains. . . . Remember how you told me that you took this short vacation right after your children had left home, and you felt you could relax so completely. Do you remember how mellow, how at ease, you felt? . . . Remember that there were no telephones . . . no televi-sion. . . no interruptions. . . . Remember that you said you could finally read a book that you'd waited so long to read. . . . You took long leisurely walks along wooded paths. . . . Remember how you described that first night when you were able to relax in your husband's (or wife's) arms. . . . Remember that time of relaxation. . . . Remember how totally relaxed you were . . . free from pressure . . . free from worries. . . .

In using a guided imagery that comes from the experience of a care receiver, we accentuate the care receiver's resources rather than our own. So, when we leave that person's room, we are not taking the resources with us; the care receiver has her own, very capable, resources still with her. Consequently, when she needs relaxation and she has no caregiver in her presence, she merely closes her eyes and returns to her own, unique place of relaxation.

AFFIRMING FREEDOM

Some caregivers—both professional and nonprofessional— tend to dictate "musts," "oughts," and "shoulds" to people in their care. And some care receivers even burden themselves with their own "musts," "oughts," and "shoulds." No matter who decrees these imperative words, they rob an individual of choices and control. When caregivers impose these words, they are controlling the people in their care rather than allowing them some control over their own lives. Some examples: "Older people must cut back on their amount of activities. . . . Terminally ill people ought to stay in bed. . . . If you have a serious illness, you should not be laughing. . . . People in their final years should want to talk about spiritual matters. . . . If someone is told that she has only a couple of years left to live, she must not smoke, ought not to drink alcohol or eat rich foods, and should not under any circumstances have sex. . . ."

By turning off our demands and by no longer imposing our views, we can prevent ourselves and those in our care from developing negative feelings about themselves and their abilities to judge for themselves what is best. Instead of limiting their choices and control of their own lives, we caregivers can consider approaches to affirming—rather than limiting—their freedom.

1. We can help them realize, and we can remind ourselves, that advanced age or illness do not affect any individual's rights. They may have fewer choices available because of an infirmity or illness, but they still have many other choices, freedoms, and rights that can be liberated from the restrictions of "must," "should," and "ought."

2. We can encourage them to challenge any statement that has a "must," "should," or "ought" in it, whether that statement is made by someone else or by themselves.

3. We can continually challenge ourselves to question any statement that contains a "must," "should," or "ought" when directed toward someone in our care.

A Plan to Eliminate Stress

When the person in our care is under stress, we can use the following seven-part outline to help uncover and ease the cause of that stress. You could give this outline to the person you are caring for to use however she wishes, or you could offer to assist her in exploring the cause of the stress and possible solutions.

1. Analyze the stress: How would you define your major stress problem? Name three or four contributing factors that cause or heighten the stress. How much time each week do you spend being aware of your

feelings connected to this problem? What will eventually happen if you do not address this problem?

2. Identify three or four possible methods of alleviating the stress connected with this problem.

3. List the advantages and disadvantages of each of the above methods.

4. Analyze these advantages and disadvantages so that you can identify the two best approaches to alleviating the stress.

5. Carefully examine the disadvantages of each of these approaches and consider how you might compensate for them.

6. Follow through with the two best approaches you have chosen.

7. Analyze the results: How are the actual results different from the expected results? What might be done to improve these results? How might the positive results be continued over time?

The person in your care will feel more control over his fate if you allow him to take the lead through this process, but if he wishes you to take the major role in this exercise it is important for you to honor that choice. The important point is to offer options, as many as possible, and then respect those he chooses.

Eliminating Self-Blaming

People who experience a great amount of illness, frailty, or debility in their final years often blame themselves for their problems: "If only I had taken better care of myself in my earlier years. . . . It's my own fault that this happened. . . . If I had been a better person. . . . God is punishing me for not being more religious. . . . I could beat this illness if only I could think more positive thoughts. . . ."

Much of this self-blaming results from irrational thinking. Such thoughts can hinder the assertion of control and decision-making that are so important at this phase of life. These irrational beliefs can be altered, however, though a shift in thought patterns. This turnaround involves changing the thought process from what is called "excessive personalization" to "reasonable depersonalization." In other words, it moves the focus from blaming oneself to more reasonable thoughts about external causes of problems. The following activity can help with this cognitive shift:

1. Ask the person in your care to make a list of various self-blaming beliefs that tend to accompany her thinking. List all the thoughts in which she blames herself for her problems. You may develop a list of five to ten self-blaming notions. It is helpful to write these down for use later in Step 3.

2. Brainstorm together about all the possible causes of her problems, causes that were or are totally out of her control. Remind her that some causes are simply unknown and that some problems occur purely by chance.

3. Go through her self-blaming list one item at a time. Ask her to make a cause-related statement that is not self-blaming, using similar vocabulary. For example, if she says, "If I would have had a more healthy diet when I was younger, I would not be so sick now," this

statement could be substituted: "People can get sick whether or not they eat healthy foods." Or, if she says, "If I only had more positive thoughts, I could get over this illness," you and she could substitute, "If positive thinking could eliminate all illness and bodily decay, optimists would never die. But optimists die of the same diseases as everyone else."

4. Suggest that your loved one or patient keep a diary of negative events. After each one, ask her to list a supposed self-centered cause, followed by a cause that is not self-centered.

5. Review the above four items with her from time to time, or whenever she seems to be falling back into a self-blaming pattern of thought. Help her recognize that external causes are of great influence on her health and welfare. Point out how these causes are often completely out of anyone's control.

CONTROL FOR THE LESS RESPONSIVE PERSON

We may incorrectly assume that people whose conditions make them appear less responsive—if they are heavily sedated, continually sleepy, or compromised by paralysis or stroke, for example—do not need or cannot exercise any control. The labeling of people as "unresponsive" or, even worse, "vegetative" can sometimes be inaccurate as well as cruel. It can be inaccurate in relation to the notion that such patients cannot hear, because several studies have shown that hearing is often the last sense to disappear. A patient may appear unaware of goings-on in his room, but he may be hearing every word that is spoken. Other studies on "near-death" experiences show that some people have a sensation of transcending their bodies before dying and peering down on their entire surroundings. "Unresponsive" people may very well see everything around them. These studies remind us to respect those in our care by imagining that they hear every word we say and may see everything we do in their presence, even if they do not appear to respond outwardly.

No matter how unresponsive they may seem, their need for a sense of control is still very important. As Avery D. Weisman has written in *The Coping Capacity*, "Even a trivial option at a propitious moment is a soft declaration of control and thus may make a significant difference."[2]

The following suggestions can foster a sense of control that can make a significant difference to less responsive patients:

1. Upon entering the room, always greet the person who is seemingly unresponsive before acknowledging anyone else.

2. Whenever in his presence, never speak about the person who appears unresponsive without speaking to him directly, regardless of his state of alertness.

3. Always react to any signal, any form of communication from him—the slight raising of a finger, blink of an eye, softest sound, turn of the head, or slightest smile.

4. Always offer him choices, or imply choices, no matter how insignificant they may seem to you or how unresponsive he may appear. If you need to turn him onto his side, for instance, first say, "I am about to move you to your right side. I hope that is okay."

Then pause to acknowledge the possibility of a response. Then and only then, move him.

5. Always look for some form of confirmation from him before initiating any change in care. Pause. Look. Listen first.

6. Thank him whenever he cooperates with you or is attentive to you. Sometimes seriously ill and dying people have only two options left in life—to cooperate or not cooperate. When they choose to cooperate, always thank them.

LETTING GO OF THE RIGHT TO BE IN CONTROL

Near the very end of life, a person has usually lost almost all threads of control and senses a need to let go, to relinquish any remaining grasp at control. At that moment, she somehow feels an appropriateness in surrendering to the dying process. But this is not a surrender in defeat. Just the opposite. Letting go of the right to be in control is another choice. A choice consciously made and exercised. An assertion of power, in fact: the ultimate exercise of power.

An ancient philosopher, Lao Tzu, saw the truth of attaining power through letting go.

> *The Way is gained by daily loss,*
> *Loss upon loss until*
> *At last comes rest.*
> *By letting go, it all gets done;*
> *The world is won by those who let it go!*

Those words can serve as a daily meditation toward the end of life, a meditation exploring choice and control in the process of letting go.

DO NOT STRAIGHTEN OUT

Caregivers sometimes succumb to the temptation of trying to "straighten out" the people in our care. We act like parents trying to mold children before they grow up and move out of our orbit. But we forget that the people in our care have grown up, lived full lives, and have the right not to be straightened out or changed to meet our desires, expectations, or values. The following exercise can help prevent us from falling victim to the temptation to straighten them out. If we must straighten out something, we can go home and clean our closets!

Before plunging ahead to tell your patient or loved one what he must do ("Have a more upbeat outlook; things could be worse," or "Work a little harder on your physical therapy," or "Just try a little harder to eat some more food."), try these steps to see whether you are in a "straightening out" mode:

1. Stop.

2. Look.

3. Listen.

4. If you feel the urge to do anything else, stop.

5. Look.

6. Listen.

7. If, once again, you feel the urge, stop.

8. Look.

9. Listen.

After this exercise, if you still feel a need to do something for or to your patient or loved one, at least ask her permission first. This will give her some measure of choice and control before you intervene.

THE CAREGIVER'S ATTITUDE

Over the years, I have suggested the following meditations for caregivers to read each day before beginning their caregiving tasks. These two meditations can help you realize the importance of allowing your care recipients the right to be in control.

I.

The sea is mightier than any river.
Yet the sea lies below any river,
Is open to any river,
And receives any river.
The caregiver of the dying represents a sea of love.

There might be an angry, rushing river.
There might be a lazy, tired river.
There might be a crooked, treacherous river.
There might be a polluted river.
The sea is open to them all.
The sea receives them all.
They are all transformed in the sea
Because the sea allows them to transform.
The caregiver of the dying represents a sea of love.

II.
People say that it is absurd to allow the dying to
have control.
People say that such an idea is impractical.
Look inside yourself.
Would you feel comfort around the person who gives
you choices,
Or the person who takes choices away from you?
Would you respect the person who trusts your
decisions,
Or the person who does not allow you to make
decisions?
Would you cheat a marathon runner out of his last
mile?
Would you take the brush away from an artist
before he makes his signature?
The caregiver has the attitude of allowing.
That is the greatest wisdom.
That is being very practical.

THE CAREGIVER'S HUMILITY

We caregivers need to relinquish our own control continually in order to facilitate choices and control for those in our care. An important prerequisite for relinquishing control is humility—the recognition of our own shortcomings and our own dependence on other people. The following activity can help us recognize this reality.

Caregiver's Self-Assessment

1. Give yourself an honest grade from A through F in each of the following commonly admired traits:
   patience
   compassion
   courage
   fidelity
   self-control
   gentleness
   love
   truthfulness
   sincerity
   friendship

2. Next to each of these traits, write the name of a friend or acquaintance who, you believe, would receive a better grade in that particular area.

3. Observe these people, and others around you, including those in your care, as necessary complements to you. Realize that we all are interdependent.

GIVER–RECEIVER DIALOGUE

Whenever you find yourself disagreeing with the actions or attitudes of your care recipients, you might find some emotional assistance by engaging in imaginary dialogues with them. If you object to your care recipient's decision not to treat her illness aggressively, for example, you could imagine her sitting in a chair across from you as you ask why she has made that choice. Imagine her likely response. An imaginary conversation would ensue and possibly help you to a better understanding of her choice.

Even if you come to no clearer an understanding or an agreement with her decision, the effort of doing this exercise can be beneficial to you in and of itself because it reinforces your desire to understand and to accept her, a major goal of good caregiving.

GETTING AWAY FROM THE CAREGIVER'S SELF-IMPOSED "MUSTS"

We considered the patients' benefits of reducing imposed "musts," "shoulds," and "oughts" on page 34. We caregivers can also benefit by diminishing the "musts" we impose on ourselves because they can inhibit our total effectiveness, create an artificial barrier between us and the people we care for, and adversely influence our sense of self-worth.

We can turn this situation around by challenging our "musts" and substituting some rationality. For instance, "I must always have a positive attitude when I am around those in my care," can be changed to "I will try to have a positive attitude if that helps them, but if I am unable to do so all the time, I am not a failure."

CHANGING THE CAREGIVER'S "I NEED" TO "I WANT"

Whether we do this consciously or unconsciously, we sometimes subtly control our care recipients by imposing our own needs on them. This diminishes their own control. We may think, "I need to have my patient appreciate everything I do. . . . I need to have this person be as cooperative with me as she is with her other caregivers. . . . I need to have my mother agree with whatever I recommend for her. . . ."

When we catch ourselves imposing our supposed needs, we reduce tension that has been building up, both in ourselves and probably in our care receivers. As we discussed earlier in regard to a patient's "needs" and "wants," we can make a similar switch here to benefit ourselves. We can reframe our supposed "needs" as "wants." And when we do substitute "want" for "need," we tend to end the sentence differently, in ways that put matters in better perspective.

Using the examples above, we can rephrase them this way: "I want my patient to appreciate everything that I do, but my world will not end if that doesn't happen. . . . I want this person to be as cooperative with me as she is with other caregivers, but I will understand if she needs to treat me differently. . . . I want my mother to agree with all my recommendations, but I will certainly survive without her compliance to my wishes. Besides, she usually knows what's best for her."

THE CAREGIVER'S REPORT CARD

After nineteen activities and exercises, you probably wonder how you are doing. At the end of each week, you can give a report card to the people in your care and ask them to grade you on an A to F range. This does turn the tables a bit. People who are seriously ill or dying often feel as though they are the ones being inspected, judged, or graded. This exercise not only gives them another opportunity to exercise some control, but it also shows you how well you are progressing as a caregiver, how much you have helped your care recipients exercise their right to a sense of control, and what may still need to be achieved. Some of the subjects in the report card that follows have not been discussed yet in this book (such as humor, touch, gentleness), but they are included here because they are appropriate items for your care recipient to evaluate.

The Caregiver's Report Card	
Subject	*Grade*
Allowing me to make my own decisions	_____
Knowing or finding answers to my questions	_____
Listening skills	_____
Appropriate touch	_____
Appropriate humor	_____
Gentleness	_____
Ability to address my physical needs	_____
Ability to address my emotional needs	_____
General comments about how my caregiver might improve:	

_____

_____

_____

From time to time, you can refer back to previous report cards to chart your progress. Do not hesitate to give yourself a gold star, a special dessert after dinner, an hour's free time to do whatever you wish—you deserve a reward for all your efforts.

CHAPTER TWO

The Right to Have a Sense of Purpose

In the last phases of life, many people lose much more than good health. They lose their accustomed roles within their families, their occupations, and their communities. When their roles are diminished or erased completely, another significant loss creeps in: a lost sense of purpose.

Throughout most adults' lives, a sense of purpose is typically linked to—and sometimes defined by—their work, family, and society. If you are an engineer, your purpose is to design efficient, durable structures. If you are a parent, your purpose is to provide for your family and raise responsible, happy children. If you are a volunteer at a neighborhood school or soup kitchen, your purpose is to give something back to your community. Our sense of purpose often makes life worth living—it's what we do, it's what we give others, it's what makes us get out of bed in the morning and gear into action.

When people can no longer participate as fully as they once did in family, work, and community life, it is easily understandable why they wonder, "What's my purpose anymore?" Yet purpose can be found. It may simply lie undiscovered in different or unusual places, and does not have to be equated with jobs or roles in family or society.

One of the first steps in finding a new sense of purpose, in fact, is to recognize that purpose does not necessarily have to be associated with a job or a role in the family or community. There are a multitude of other avenues leading toward a sense of purpose. It can be found in making a positive difference in others' lives, in redirecting one's life toward new goals, in doing things we always wanted to do. A new sense of direction can be forged by looking at our final years as a time of challenge rather than a time of retreat, as we learned from Gary's story in the Introduction. Or a new sense of purpose may be created by withdrawing from external matters in order to put our internal house in order.

I begin this chapter's series of anecdotes with Albert because his story shows how a sense of purpose can be unearthed by digging into the past. Caregivers who work with elderly people often call this a "life review tool." By recalling past experiences—moments of feeling proud or feeling loved, for example—an older person can recapture some of the same feelings for the present. These recollections can recharge an old sense of purpose. That is what happened with Albert.

Albert

Hospice workers had labeled Albert "nonresponsive." I had visited him twice, but he had not acknowledged me in any way. I might as well have been invisible. On my third visit, I didn't expect any difference in his response, but I went anyway. I noticed a book on his bedside table and remembered that it had been there, in the exact same spot, during both my visits in the past two weeks.

I sat down next to his bed. He didn't move, look at me, or say a word. I picked up the book and flipped through it. It was a history of black baseball leagues. Suddenly I heard Albert grunting quietly. It was the first sound I'd heard from him. His eyes opened. He grunted again and, with his eyes, he directed me toward his right hand. He was holding up three fingers, then two fingers. He paused. Again he held up three fingers, then two. His eyes went to the book in my hands. I realized that Albert wanted me to turn to page 32 in the book. I did. There was a photograph of a young man named Albert, nicknamed "Speedball."

I looked at him and asked, "Speedball?"

He grunted, nodded, and smiled all in one movement. Then, still smiling, he closed his eyes.

This still, quiet, "nonresponsive" man contained within himself the knowledge that he had once been a formidable athlete, that he would always be to himself the vibrant handsome youth known as "Speedball."

"Did you know Satchell Paige?" I asked.

Another grunt, a nod, an even broader smile.

We had begun a dialogue. An identity was discovered. Albert's purpose had been found. His realization that I knew his past purpose was giving him a sense of purpose in the present.

You will recall my "stop—look—and listen" exercise. If I had not consciously done that and taken the time to look, pause, and take stock of simply the ordinary surroundings in Albert's room, I never would have discovered this crucial part of his identity, one that would become the start of a very positive, life-affirming, life review.

Life review techniques may also reveal material that can prevent people from finding a sense of purpose in the present. People can get stuck in the past, hung up on an event or person that keeps them from functioning as fully as they can in the present and future. To help them move on to be able to exercise their right to a sense of purpose, we caregivers need to help them get unstuck from the past. Such was the situation with Amanda.

Amanda

At age 60, Amanda was suffering from lung cancer with brain metastasis. Whenever she was asked about her feelings, she replied with tears in her eyes, "I feel angry and cheated."

When I first heard her say this, I did not automatically assume that she was referring directly to her terminal illness. As we continued to talk, she revealed that her feelings of anger and injustice stemmed from her failure years ago to end a marriage when she discovered that her husband had been having an affair for seven years. Instead of leaving him then, she had stayed with him for another eight years as he continued the affair. Eventually they divorced. Amanda's feelings were not caused by a sense of her future being wasted, but by a sense of her past being wasted.

Amanda decided that she could not address her future until she first addressed her past. She decided to telephone her ex-husband to tell him how despicable he was for the way he treated her. This decision was quite out of character with her normally meek nature. She asked me to be with her in a supportive role when she placed the phone call.

I did stay with her but she hardly needed me there. Her meekness evaporated and she became the person I later came to call "Amanda the Hun." Oh, she was good! The process of confronting her past was wonderful for her—it freed her. Unstuck from her past, Amanda was now able to devote her energy to her present and future.

Linda

As Linda entered the last few months of her life, the physical characteristics of her illness were dramatic reminders of a psychological and physical event from her past. Her story is one of immense courage, as she not only confronted her past but also transformed her courage into a sense of purpose for the present and future.

At age 44, Linda had cancer of the uterus with metastasis to her spinal cord and subsequent paraplegia from her mid-breast downward. When I met her for an initial interview and assessment, she volunteered that she had been sexually abused when she was four years old by a teenage babysitter. The incident was still of major significance to her after forty years. She revealed this history before she even mentioned other important concerns of the present, such as the emotional state of her three young children, her own feelings about her debilitation, or her worries about her husband's welfare. Linda's childhood nightmare was crying out to be confronted and explored immediately. She needed to discuss it before she could address all the other issues associated with her imminent death.

Unveiling that 40-year-old trauma was frightening for Linda because she had previously told only her husband. But after revealing all the details to me, Linda experienced a sense of great *relief. She felt a colossal burden had started to lift. Telling her story was so therapeutic that she decided to tell others, first her children and then her friends. As she told them one at a time, even more of the burden was lifted. She even invited members of her church prayer group to visit her and hear her story. With each of these meetings, Linda gave her listeners an emphatic charge: Do your best to end the horrors of sexual abuse in whatever way you can. That charge was particularly powerful because it came from Linda, only a few weeks away from death, and it was her last attempt to create a purpose in her life.*

People facing death often have a profound desire to feel that they are still part of the world of the living. They don't want to be counted out just yet. They want to be heard and appreciated for what they can give to others. They want their lives to have meaning and purpose. Death may be on the horizon, but they do lead a life, though that life may have changed direction and form. As caregivers, we need to remind ourselves repeatedly never to forget that a dying person is a living person. We can use the following techniques to help them maintain a sense of purpose even though that purpose may change near life's end.

Tools and techniques for promoting the right to have a sense of purpose

THE MEDICINE MAN

This guided imagery exercise[3] can help sick and dying people reach within themselves to pull out strengths and resources they may not realize they possess. I am convinced that we all have within ourselves our own doctor, social worker, psychologist, and spiritual advisor. As caregivers, we can try to help those in our care get in touch with their own "in-house" helpers. For this exercise, the caregiver may lead the imagery narrative in your own voice or record it for your patients or loved ones to use whenever they wish.

The exercise here involves an imagined meeting with a medicine man. However, the specifics of this wise individual can be adapted to what will be comfortable to the care recipient. Instead of a medicine man, the individual may be a Tibetan monk, or a wise woman, for example. The discussion that takes place and the role-playing are the key elements that can make this a very successful exercise.

THE MEDICINE MAN

Close your eyes and imagine that you have heard about a very unusual medicine man, a great medicine man who knows the secret of finding purpose in our final years. You have decided to go and talk to him to find out what main purpose you have set before you between now and the end of your life.

To meet this medicine man, you have flown by helicopter to the top of a mountain in a deserted part of New Mexico. You find yourself seated at a campfire and he is sitting across from you. You can barely make out his features. Imagine what he is wearing. . . . How does his body appear? . . . Examine his face closely. . . . Look into his all-knowing eyes.

continued

Now ask him what important task you are to accomplish between now and the end of your life. . . . At first, the medicine man just stares at you in silence. . . . His eyes penetrate into the depths of your being. You watch him watching you. . . . Finally he speaks, telling you what to do. What does he say about your purpose during the remainder of your life? . . . What does the medicine man say is your goal during your final days on this earth? . . .

Now imagine yourself as the medicine man. . . . What does it feel like to be him? . . . What feelings do you have toward the person sitting across from you? . . . What do you want to say and do for this person? . . .

Become yourself again and respond to this medicine man. How do you react to what has just been said to you? . . . What feelings do you have toward the medicine man? . . .

Once again, imagine becoming the medicine man. Is there anything else you need to say to the person who has come to visit you? . . .

As yourself again, get ready to leave the medicine man. . . . How do you wish to say good-bye? . . . Say good-bye to him in whatever manner seems most fitting to you. . . .

Slowly open your eyes. . . . We can now, if you wish, talk about what you have just experienced.

RANDOM ACTS OF KINDNESS

Caregivers can suggest the following activities to help car recipients regain a sense of self-worth, meaning, and purpose.

You can suggest one, two, or three and let the person in your care decide which seems most appropriate. You may want to join in and if you do, you will find your own sense of purpose can also increase. These activities may not be for everyone, however. All require some energy that may not be available to every care recipient. If you find nothing here that your care recipient wants to do, or is able to do, you might jointly come up with other activities that are easier to do. But hopefully, this list will spark some creative ideas.

1. Make some cookies and lemonade and give them away to neighbors.

2. Go to a nursing home and visit someone who never receives visitors.

3. Go to a playground and pass out free balloons to children or flowers to adults on the street.

4. Be a sounding board for another person. Listen to someone else for an hour without saying the word "I."

5. Make a conscious effort to compliment people. Their appreciation will come back to you as immediate good feelings.

In the Affirmative

We've seen in chapter 1 how affirmations can enhance a person's sense of control. Affirmations can also promote a sense of purpose when used to restate desires as realities. Instead of saying, "I wish that my pain would go away," a person could state this in the affirmative by rephrasing it, "I am free from pain."

Now move to affirmations that reflect wishes, dreams, and hopes—truths in the making. Stating something is a step toward making it happen. Follow each affirmation with this statement: "I am now in the process of creating this reality or a better reality," or "I am now in the process of making this happen."

1. Ask the person in your care to write an affirmation—a present desire as a present reality—so that it can be read each evening before bed or each morning upon waking.

2. Ask the person to visualize the affirmation with every possible detail happening in the present moment.

3. Post the written affirmation in several locations—on mirrors, refrigerator doors, bedposts—so that it is constantly in sight.

4. For even greater effect, ask the person in your care to write the affirmation ten times using the pronoun "I." ("I, Doug, am free from pain.") Then have him write it ten times using "You." ("You, Doug, are free from pain.") Finally, bring it home as a flat-out declaration of objective fact: "Doug is free from pain."

PARADIGM SHIFT

Although "paradigm shift" has become one of the great intellectual cliches of the late twentieth century, it can be a useful way to describe the process of tearing down an existing framework and reassembling the pieces into something new and quite different. The aging process often requires people to make "paradigm shifts" in their sense of purpose and meaning, as well as in other aspects of their lives. In our caregiving work, we can help them look at the traditional definition of purpose and redefine it to suit their needs when they are ill or nearing the end of life. The following story, adapted from an old parable, can serve as a subject of meditation or used as a discussion to help people begin to make this paradigm shift in their minds and attitudes.

The Tale of the Sands

In a far-off land, a stream gains strength as it rushes down a mountainside. It passes around and through various obstacles as it finally makes its way to the sands of a desert. Just as it has managed to move past every rock, fallen tree, and other barrier, the stream tries to cross the desert. But as rapidly as it runs into the desert, it disappears just as fast.

Embedded in the memory of the stream is the fact that it has crossed the desert at another time. That memory takes the form of an internal voice, whispering, "The wind can cross the desert, and so can the stream."

The voice puzzles the stream at first because the stream cannot understand how the wind's ability to fly has anything to do with the stream. The stream feels that it can only continue to be absorbed by the desert sands because streams are always confined to the ground. But the internal voice persists, "Choose not to be absorbed by the sand. Choose to fly like

continued

the wind. The wind will help get you across the desert."

The stream protests. After all, it feels that it has always served the purpose of rushing across objects, rushing around or through whatever gets in its path. Why would the stream have to change its ways? Why would it want to lose its accustomed individuality?

Then a voice appears to come from the sand itself. "Trust the wind. It has carried you in previous times. Trust the wind. If you do not trust the wind, you will only become a quagmire."

The stream protests, "Why can I not just remain a stream?"

"That is not even a choice," a voice responds, "Trust the wind or become a quagmire. Trust the wind."

Somehow that voice seems distantly familiar to the stream. There is a faint remembrance that the stream was not always a stream, and a realization that it definitely had a beginning elsewhere. The stream vaguely remembers being held in the arms of the wind. It recalls a lighter state, a state of freedom.

Finally the stream is convinced that it needs to trust the wind. Raising its vapor into the welcoming arms of the wind, the stream experiences itself being carried gently above the sands. Gently carried to the top of a distant mountain, gently being released by the wind—to once again become a stream. Thus by letting go of the familiar does the stream finally achieve its real purpose.

Like the stream in the parable, we occasionally need to let go of past expectations to be transformed. We need to let go in trust. Meditation on the parable can help someone near the end of life shift many paradigms. Making these shifts helps prepare them for the final shift from life to death.

CHANGING PHILOSOPHY

"I am old and therefore useless. . . . No one in this nursing home cares about me. . . . God must not love me if I'm allowed to become so ill. . . ."

How often have we heard negative statements like these? It is not uncommon for people to develop distressing beliefs in their final years. One way caregivers can help is to identify and write down one of the patient's major views that upsets both your care recipient and/or her families and friends. Then discuss various ways that this philosophy is expressed, both consciously and subconsciously, in everyday activities. Does she complain openly, or does she sulk about her state of health, for example? Has she lost interest in friends, food, activities, or other things that used to hold her interest?

Then you can help her develop alternate, more positive viewpoints and write them down for her as a reminder. Whatever the new viewpoint entails, it will most likely succeed if it makes some logical sense, is practical, and allows for flexibility. An example:

Old philosophy: "I'm old and therefore useless."

New philosophy: "I am old, but that doesn't have to have a bearing on whether I am useful or useless. Many older people have been quite useful to society. The same is true of young people. There is no direct correlation between age and usefulness."

Caregivers can guide those in their care to look for ways to make this new philosophical position a reality. Perhaps notes can be taken to show how the new position would improve the person's environment. Each of the following areas can be examined:

Relations with spouse or partner

Relations with children

Relations with members of the opposite sex

Relations with members of the same sex

Physical health

Attitudes toward change

Attitudes toward religious/spiritual issues

Responses to criticism and rejection from others

Responses to progressive physical deterioration

Responses to the imminence of death

Simply stating a new point of view will not be enough to really effect a change. Caregivers need to reinforce the point that simply examining a new philosophy is not as beneficial as actually adapting and manifesting it. Together, caregiver and receiver can map out a step-by-step plan to put the new, healthier philosophy into practice.

LATE-LIFE CRISIS

A midlife crisis is well recognized, along with the changes it may bring. We may wear new clothing, change hair styles or color, adopt a new political cause, go back to school, find different friends—or even change jobs, leave a spouse, or move to another home. While many jokes are made about midlife crises, they can give a person a new sense of energy, a new purpose.

What about a late-life crisis? When major reassessment occurs later in life, we still may make many changes. People in their later years can study for a high school equivalency exam or enroll in a college course. They can join a political interest group, start a stock investment club, or develop a new hobby. If they've worn conservative blues and grays, they may enjoy trying neon orange shirts and lime green slacks!

Psychologically, spiritually, and socially, some elderly or ill people may be too quick to believe they no longer have any purpose in living. Yet they can be helped to discover new purposes. Caregivers can encourage them to try one, two, or several activities, such as those suggested above, to introduce new experiences and purposes into their lives, to move them out of stagnant, unsatisfying routines that lack any taste, exploration, or excitement or the fun of trying something new.

LOOKING FORWARD TO TOMORROW

A sense of purpose can oftentimes be found in simply knowing that there is a place for us in tomorrow's agenda. Positive anticipation about tomorrow is an inherent part of having—and maintaining—a sense of purpose. Caregivers can foster that feeling of positive anticipation in small but significant ways, such as bringing something new for care recipients to enjoy at regular intervals. These efforts need not be costly or time-consuming, but they will let patients and loved ones know that they have a place on your agenda tomorrow, and that is something to look forward to. Here are some suggestions for things you could do regularly:

- Give them a different greeting card each Monday
- Read a chapter of a book to them each day
- Treat them to a surprise flavor of ice cream every Friday
- Play a different music record, tape, or CD each week
- Bring a different video to watch every Wednesday

APPRECIATION AWARD

Social workers, nurses, and other caregivers are honored annually for their specific contributions: Social Worker Month, Nursing Week, Volunteer Appreciation Day. Why not have a time set aside to show appreciation to patients? Most caregivers readily acknowledge that they receive immense benefits from their patients, but there is not an officially recognized month, week, or even day for them.

Caregiving teams could correct this oversight by presenting a plaque, or a bouquet, or a single rose to a care recipient. Every care recipient would have a special day when everyone on the caregiving team would somehow show extra appreciation for that person: Bertha's Day, Andrew's Day, Shirley's Day. Such recognition would acknowledge the gifts that have been received from that individual. This gesture has several benefits: It not only honors the recipient and makes him aware that, even in illness, an individual can give to others, but it also reminds us that we are helped by those we help. Care is a two-way street. Gifts travel in both directions between caregiver and the people in our care.

PASS IT ON

Various forms of "life review" can clarify a person's sense of purpose. The following life review activity is intended to aid ill and dying people by helping them to look back on what they have learned over the years so that those lessons can be passed to others. Meaning is borrowed from the past to lend meaning to the present and future. The activity offers incomplete sentences for your care recipient to complete.

My Life's Purpose

1. I feel people need to cherish _____ most in life.

2. The best thing people can do with their lives, in my opinion, is _____.

3. My formula for getting lots of fun out of life is _____.

4. I have found that friendships work if people are willing to _____.

5. I have found that the secret to feeling content at the end of the day is_____.

6. What I want people to learn most from my last years on this earth is_____.

7. The one thing for which I most want to be remembered is _____.

This activity could be followed by a discussion between caregiver and your patient or loved one, a discussion about how your care recipient might pass on this knowledge to relatives, friends, or others. The activity of reaching into the past to complete those sentences often helps to uncover a purpose in the past. The follow-up discussion can help transfer that purpose into the future.

A SIMPLE LIFE REVIEW

Two ingredients are essential to a successful life review when someone is nearing the end of life: brevity and emphasis on the positive. In the following life review, caregivers can help those in their care look at past and recent purposes. All these questions, or only a few, may be used.

1. When you look back on your life and think about the really fun moments, what comes to mind?

2. What past occasion do you remember that generated the feeling of being proud? Describe what happened.

3. At what moment in your life were you most aware of the meaning of the word "love?" Elaborate.

4. If there was one event that you would like to relive, what would it be? Describe what happened.

5. How would you describe your "good old days?" Elaborate.

6. In the remaining time in your life, what do you want most to accomplish?

Although this activity emphasizes the positive, an opportunity to uncover negative events could also be provided if such events are hindering someone from moving toward the future with full attention. If you feel that might be the case, you could add another question to those above: "What event in your past causes you still to feel some anger? Describe what happened." Emphasizing the positive may be most appreciated, but we would be doing a disservice to people in our care if we do not give them an opportunity to discuss and free themselves from past negative events as well.

SINGLE-RECOLLECTION LIFE REVIEW

Another way to do a life review exercise is to ask a single question: "What one memory stands out from either first or second grade?" This simple question can elicit a great deal of information. When we cast our memory back that long ago, whatever memory we recapture must have some significance. It was significant then, and it still has some significance now. That single memory can reveal much information about someone.

Here is my personal example: The sharpest memory I have from first grade is walking to school in Orlando, Florida. A block from home, I heard a girl screaming in her backyard. I ran toward the sound and saw a three- or four-year-old girl, standing on the seat of a swing and pointing to a garter snake in the grass below. I found a forked twig on the ground and pinned the snake, so she could jump off the swing and run into her house.

Why do I still remember that brief event so vividly? As I've thought about it, I came up with three possible explanations. My father was a very macho guy. The significance of this save-the-damsel-in-distress rescue could be that I knew my dad would be very pleased by my actions, and I always wanted to please him. Another reason could be that this was the first time I earned respect from someone of the opposite sex— and possibly the only time I assuredly did. It would have satisfied my need to be appreciated by women. And the third explanation for the strength and clarity of this memory could be that I was clearly able to help someone in need. The desire to help people in need has been constant throughout my adult life; every occupation I have ever had can be called a "helping profession." All three possible explanations, taken together, say a great deal about who I am, what I value, and how I see my sense of purpose.

If you do this single-recollection life review exercise with someone who recalls a negative memory, do not think it is misguided or useless. Sometimes negative memories can have a positive influence. If, for example, the person in your care remembers his first-grade teacher asking a question that he couldn't answer, that little boy may have grown up reading and studying ever since, always being prepared so he will not be embarrassed again.

What the Teacher Says

Our early teachers often have a dramatic influence on us as we mature. Caregivers can take advantage of this fact by leading care recipients through the next activity, which can help those care recipients use a positive influence from the past to influence their present sense of purpose.

Ask the person in your care to recall a favorite teacher. Then inquire how that teacher would advise you on the following issues:

- How you are interacting with your family right now?
- How you spent your time last month?
- How you act when you are depressed?
- What you need to be doing with the rest of your life?

PHOTOGRAPHIC LIFE REVIEW

Family photographs are another vehicle that can help bring a past sense of purpose into the present. Caregivers can ask care receivers to choose six to eight family photographs that each represent an important chapter in their lives. Ask them to provide a narrative for each photo, including: who is in the picture, what is the occasion, what is the significance of the photograph? As caregiver, you can simply first listen to the narrative and then, perhaps, go on to explore other topics that can emerge from both what is said and what is not said, such as:

- What key family members are not present in any of these photos?
- Is more time spent with some photos and less with others?
- Are there common themes to all these photographs?
- Is there a particular significance in the locations where the photos were taken?
- Are key periods in the person's life missing in the photos selected?
- Who took the photographs?

This photographic life review should not be rushed. You may want to give the person in your care a week or two to decide which photographs to use in this activity. The process of looking over and selecting the photos can be an enjoyable learning experience in itself. It may also call to mind other photographs, family albums, or family documents that have meaning to the person in your care. Retrieving some of these from other family members or sources may open up entirely new areas of interest.

RECORDING A MESSAGE

If it seems appropriate, you may want to encourage your patient or loved one to leave some messages for posterity. A message could be written, tape-recorded, or videotaped for relatives and friends. It might include feelings, thoughts, or desires that have not been expressed previously. It could be given to relatives and friends before or after their loved one's death, as he or she prefers.

YOUR LIFE IN REVIEW

Many of us see ourselves through the eyes of other people. The way they view us may influence how we see ourselves. The same can be true for a sense of purpose. How we perceive our purpose may be closely tied to how others see it.

The following life review exercise differs from many of the other life reviews we have discussed. This activity is done for people receiving care rather than by them. It gathers other people's impressions and holds them up as a mirror for a seriously ill or dying person to consider. The information may not be as accurate as someone's own self-reported life review, but it can offer substantial pleasure, since such actions tend to focus on positive, uplifting moments.

Family, friends, and/or professional caregivers can perform this life review using one or more of the following approaches:

- Various people from the care recipient's past could offer remembrances of special moments they have shared. This can be done in person or through letters, phone calls, audiotapes, or videotapes.

- Several people could present a short history of key events and accomplishments in the person's life.

- Remembrances and recollections in the form of poetry, music, or artworks are a very special, imaginative way to give the person something completely unique as a tribute.

Whatever form the life review done by others takes, it has been my experience that this activity is an especially meaningful one for all involved, one that has the potential to foster an entirely new kind of connectedness with those we love.

CARING GUIDELINES

Our goal as caregivers is to maximize a sense of purpose for the people in our care. To reach that goal, we can incorporate the following steps in our daily care routine:

1. Realize that an individual's quality of life can only be judged by that person. We caregivers can easily impose our standards on them, but we would do them much more good if we accepted their definitions of quality of life, not ours.

2. Promote choices whenever possible. The more choices, the better. The opportunity to make choices is important to a sense of purpose because it enables an individual to be an active participant in determining his fate. And that participation is a prerequisite to knowing that his actions can make a positive difference in his life.

3. Eliminate all language, attitudes, or actions that promote stereotypes of helplessness. We caregivers should not communicate in any way that our patients' or loved ones' sense of purpose has diminished because they are ill or nearing death. Even on the last day of life, a person can have a profound purpose.

4. Allow care recipients opportunities to modify any unrealistic expectations that have been placed on them by others or by themselves. The processes of aging and dying often alter people's physical or mental capabilities. Care recipients may want caregivers to adjust our attitudes to match their adjusted capabilities. Talk about this together so that you are both in agreement about what is realistic under their present circumstances.

5. Help those in your care enjoy successful experiences, but let them define success. Normally we caregivers might think of success in terms of academic degrees, job promotions, or raises, but we could help those in our care by broadening our notions of success. Remembering something that was long forgotten, doing a task without someone else's help, or sharing

humor in the midst of trying circumstances could be examples of success for those in your care.

6. Try to establish a supportive relationship with those in your care and encourage other supportive relationships. Caregivers can be both helpers and friends when helpers and friends are wanted, but we can attempt to enlarge that circle of support by finding other helpers and friends if they are wanted.

CHAPTER THREE

The Right to Know the Truth

In a 1990 survey, I asked directors of hospices around the country to describe ideal environments for dying people, their families, and their principal caregivers. One question asked was whether dying people preferred to hear the truth, however painful, or whether they preferred to be protected from it. The results were clear-cut: 96 percent of the respondents reported that individuals near death preferred to hear the truth.

If the people in our care demand the right to know the truth, those of us around them in their final days and months need to have a system that encourages and supports that right. An open, truthful sharing of facts between caregivers and patients can create an atmosphere of trust and teamwork for all involved. It promotes a collegial relationship—one in which everyone is working together to provide the best care.

Many people who have worked in hospices attest to the value of truthfulness for both patient and caregiver. Dying patients have expressed the belief that it is easier to die when the people around them talk freely about what is going on, even if great pain and sadness accompany that honesty.

Family members who show their grief openly are also expressing their love openly. The longer we postpone facing death and the more we ignore it, the greater hold our fears have on us—the dying person as well as relatives, friends, and caregivers. The more we try to run from our fears, or pretend they don't haunt us, the more frightening and overpowering they grow.

For most of us, the unknown is ominous. Some of us try to convince ourselves that no news is good news, when we really fear the worst. But in truth, knowing is less painful than not knowing. The quality of our lives is diminished when the truth is not recognized and spoken. For people who are seriously ill or dying, there is little quality to life at all if they are deprived of the right to know the truth. But knowing the truth can enhance that quality, as Glenda's story reveals.

Glenda

Glenda knew her death was not far off. At age 85, she had chronic, obstructive pulmonary disease, and her mobility was quite limited. She needed a walker to get around her small apartment. But she wanted to remain as independent as possible and to know absolutely everything about what was going to happen to her. She peppered her doctors and nurses with questions about every possible detail of her future. She talked convincingly about adjusting to any adversity that might arise. Glenda asked her nurse, for example, about the possibility that she would eventually be unable to use her walker. The nurse confirmed that it was probable that she would soon become unable to use it.

When the nurse arrived the next day, she found Glenda crawling around the floor on hands and knees.

"What are you doing, Glenda?"

"I'm preparing myself for the future," Glenda replied with a big smile. "You know, I think I'll be ready when the time comes to get rid of the walker."

Glenda conquered a fear of the future by asking to hear the truth, pondering it, and then preparing for its consequences. This not only reduced her fears, but also increased her sense of control and sense of purpose. The truth set her free to experience a certain joy in facing the truth and satisfaction in figuring out a way to adjust to it.

Vicky

Vicky had never witnessed anyone's death. When she learned that another hospice resident was dying in the day room, she wanted to see the process firsthand. She reached for her walker and made her way down the hall. After asking the gathered family for permission to be there, she sat down to watch.

Death arrived late that afternoon, and Vicky saw everything. When a staff member suggested that she might want to leave before the funeral home people arrived, Vicky insisted on staying. She wanted to see everything that would happen. She sat quietly and watched as the body was wrapped up, strapped to a cart, and wheeled away. She watched through a window as the hearse pulled away.

Back in her own room later, Vicky said she felt better about awaiting her own death because she now knew what would happen when she died.

Death is an unknown to all of us. The journey toward it is usually fraught with numerous uncertainties that cause frightening, unnerving feelings. But we can reduce these feelings by telling a readily available truth. The people in our care have a right to hear and know that truth when they ask.

Tools and techniques for promoting the right to know the truth

ASSERTING THE RIGHT TO TRUTH

Most patients need to be more assertive because the truth is not often readily volunteered by medical professionals. Caregivers can therefore give the following suggestions to their patients to help them assert their right to hear the truth.

- Ask your physician to explain your condition fully and in terms you can understand. If you don't know a term or understand an explanation, ask the doctor to translate it into layman's language.

- Inquire about all the alternatives that may be available to treat your condition; be sure to ask about any alternatives to drugs or surgery.

- Ask about potential side-effects of any drugs that you are currently using, as well as any drugs that are suggested to you.

- Verify what your doctor says by seeking opinions from other physicians or publications.

- Before allowing a doctor to perform any procedure on you, ask about his or her past experience in doing the same procedure. Inquire about all possible complications that could result from the procedure and about the probable length of recovery time.

• Tell the physician your opinion about your condition. You know how you feel. You know your body. The doctor knows some truths, but so do you.

• Do not give your consent for any procedure until everything has been explained to your satisfaction.

PAST EXPERIENCES AND PRESENT THOUGHTS

Our past experiences tend to have a strong influence on our present thoughts. That influence is most powerful when prior experiences were laden with strong emotions. Past experiences with dying and death often mold our current ideas about the end of life.

Caregivers can help loved ones and patients deal with the reality of their present condition and the future by encouraging a discussion of former experiences that relate to their current thinking regarding death and dying. The discussion could begin by looking back on the details of the person's first encounter with death. Who was the first person they knew who died—a grandparent, parent, or neighbor? How old were they at the time? How did they cope with that death? Ask the person in your care to tell that story in the first person, present tense, as though it were happening today.

Continue the discussion by recalling other encounters with death. Are some of the same thoughts and feelings about those past deaths still present? Is there a similarity in coping styles between then and now? You could talk about what bearing this discussion has on the patient's quest for truth. Do those prior experiences cloud perceptions of present reality? Are they part of the present reality? How can this knowledge about the relationship between past and present help to sort out what is true and what is not? How does the past–present relationship help in adjusting to the future?

Once the patient has thoroughly examined how she has carried earlier experiences and feelings into the present, she may be able to see how they influence her perception of current situations. Likewise, this will help her understand how caregivers might display different attitudes because they have been influenced by their own specific past experiences. For instance, a doctor's way of interacting may well be influenced by his prior relationships with other patients. Experiences from his past might keep him from being totally honest with a patient. Conversely, former experiences might cause a social worker to overemphasize the positives, or experiences from a nurse's past might cause him to emphasize the negatives. All too often, past family experiences can cause a relative to want to protect a loved one from painful truths, but this may actually be doing the loved one a disservice.

By considering questions such as these, a caregiver can see how a patient's quest for truth can often be complicated by many variables, including past experiences that influence the present. Yet a thoughtful examination of prior influences—by both the person receiving care as well as various caregivers—can move the patient ahead in that journey toward the truth.

THOUGHTS: HINDERING AND HELPFUL

This exercise helps untangle two different paths in the quest for truth. It helps patients examine internal messages that arise when depression and pain are at their worst. During those moments, some of these internal messages are not completely truthful because they are overburdened with emotional overtones and value judgments.

Caregivers can assist by guiding a discussion of "hindering thoughts" and "helpful thoughts." Ask the person in your care to examine the hindering thoughts in the left column and compare them with the helpful thoughts opposite them on the right. Are these thoughts similar in any way? This can be followed by a discussion about ways to alter the unhelpful thoughts.

Hindering Thoughts	*Helpful Thoughts*
People never do exactly what I want them to do.	I will just have to live with that.
A poor health system has caused my problems.	I do not help my situation by blaming others.
It's not fair that I am in so much pain.	What can I learn from this situation?
My caregiver is not entertaining for me.	If I cannot change her, I will learn to accept her.

This exercise helps patients sort out how they think and why. When they reach this understanding, they may also gain a better grasp of others' thinking and communication. This knowledge is one more step toward the truth, toward separating what is true and what is not, what is objective and what is laden with emotional overtones and value judgments. And most importantly, it represents a movement away from negativity and toxic thoughts to positive, constructive ones.

COUNTERING IRRATIONALITY

"Counters" are thoughts or activities that can stop untrue ideas in their tracks. Sometimes humorous, counters act as a red light to irrational thoughts that are starting to spin out of control. A single word like "Nonsense!" or "Hogwash!" is an example of a counter. When an irrational thought begins, "My life is over . . . ," it can be interrupted with a counter: "Nonsense! Nothing but nonsense!" Or it can be stopped with a sentence: "Nobody's life is over until it's over."

Caregivers can help those in their care construct forceful counters for stopping irrational thoughts so they can move instead in a more rational, logical direction. Here are some useful tips.

- Counters need to stop irrational thinking abruptly in order to be effective. Make them short and punchy, like "Hogwash!" Say them as soon as the irrational thought arises.

- The best counters are those suggested by the patient, not the caregiver.

- Write down these counters. The more the better.

- Develop several forms of counters: words, phrases, sentences, philosophical arguments; the greater the variety, the better. Consult a thesaurus if need be.

- Suggest practicing these counters aloud whenever an irrational thought comes to mind. Practice some more, as long as the irrational thoughts recur.

In using any of the activities in this book, caregivers need to remember that they help only people who want to be helped. It is particularly relevant to keep that in mind with this counter technique. We might call a thought "irrational," but our loved ones or patients might not. If they do not want to be helped in finding "more rational" thoughts, we must accept them for who they are and what they think. And it is entirely possible that their "irrational thought" serves a positive purpose, as seen in chapter 1. Their thought may be a way of exercising control or achieving a purpose known only to them. So, as with all exercises suggested on these pages, our caregivers' goals must be compatible with care recipients' goals. We cannot force our views, methods, or judgments on them.

GETTING AT THE FREEDOM OF TRUTH

"The truth shall set you free." Those words are often spoken, but how is their meaning made real? How can we help our care recipients gain the freedom that comes from knowing the truth? The six questions in this exercise are aimed at discovering the truth within oneself. Caregivers can provide these questions in written form for loved ones or patients to use at their leisure, or they can be discussed together during a visit. If you do have a conversation about them, you can enrich the experience for both of you if you admit and explore your own irrational thinking.

Discovering the Truth to Set You Free

1. What belief do I want to dispute and surrender? (That belief could be considered "irrational," such as "I must be physically attractive and healthy in order to be loved by anyone.")
2. Is it possible for me to support this belief rationally?
3. What evidence might support the truth of this belief?
4. What evidence might support the falseness of this belief?
5. What is the worst possible thing that could happen to me if this belief is, in fact, true?
6. What value do I have in my life even if this belief is true?

After exploring these questions honestly, many people discover that their beliefs had little or no basis. The result of that discovery is a great freedom from past fears, hurts, anger, or depression. Even when some truth does play a role in one of those fears or hurts, it is really not so terrible. There is a gain in perspective. In spite of fears, hurts, anger, and depression, people discover that there is still much of value in life. Realizing this can free them to think and act more rationally.

SPEAKING OF PAIN

For most people in our care, much of their time is dominated by feelings and thoughts connected to pain. In their desire for the truth, they may want to examine and clarify this relationship with pain. The following activity could assist in that process.

1. Ask him to close his eyes and focus on the area of his body that is producing the greatest amount of pain.

2. Ask him to imagine that this painful area is a person. With pen and paper, he could answer the following questions, or he could tell you his answers and you could write them for him:

> What name would you give this person (pain)?
> When was this person born and under what circumstances?
> Write a short history of how this person grew.
> What have been the high points and low points of this person's life?

3. Then ask him to write, or dictate to you, a conversation that he might have with this person (pain), addressing the following questions:

> What do you want to say to this person?
> How does this person respond?
> What do you then say?

Encourage him to expand the conversation, going back and forth with questions and answers to discover what can be learned about his relationship to pain. Finally, suggest that he write (or dictate) a summary of what has been learned through this activity.

DISCOVERING THE SUBJECTIVE TRUTH

Truth can be subjective as well as objective. A subjective truth can often have more influence than an objective truth. A particular stimulus, for example, could cause intolerable pain for one person but only mild pain for another. Each level of pain is true for the individual who is subjectively feeling it.

A Sufi saying acknowledges the subjectivity of truth:

A king can want more when he has a vast kingdom,
and ten Sufis can feel warm under a single blanket.

Subjective attitudes can transform a single objective reality into several possible subjective truths.

The following activity offers a way to transform the objective reality of intense pain into the truth of subjectively manageable pain.

1. Help the person in your care enter a state of relaxation, either through concentrating, breathing, or calming verbal assurances.

2. Suggest that she scan her body mentally and identify an area that is experiencing pain.

3. Ask her to identify a color that she considers soothing and peaceful.

4. Suggest that she imagine that color encircling and permeating the painful area, that she visualize and feel the color bringing comfort and health to that area.

5. Ask her to concentrate on breathing, with each exhalation marking an increase in the color's vividness and strength.

6. Suggest that she visualize and feel the area as very relaxed and filled with healthy energy.

This exercise could result in the changing of the physical truth of pain into the mental truth of a calming, energizing force field of color and vitality.

THE GRASS CAN SOMETIMES BE BROWNER

People approaching death often feel cheated out of life. They ask, "Why me? . . . Why now? . . . Why couldn't I have gotten a warning? . . . Couldn't I just be given ten more years, or even ten more months?" Frequently accompanying this feeling of being cheated, is a fantasy about having a better existence than the current one, a feeling that they would be so much better "if only. . . ."

The message of the next activity is simply to help the patient experience what we know to be true, but often forget: "The fantasy may not always be that wonderful, and the reality may not be as bad as I have painted it." The intention here is to help people examine their true state, which they may discover is not all that bad. They may in fact, come to see negatives in their fantasy world and positives in their real world.

1. Ask your loved ones or patients to make a detailed list of all the elements in their fantasy world. For example, "I would have no aches and pains. . . . I would not age. . . . I would be able to eat anything I wanted, go anywhere I wanted to go. . . ."

2. Tell them to close their eyes and imagine that all the elements of the fantasy came true. Imagine that this fantasy world will last forever, that nothing will ever diminish or destroy it.

3. Encourage them to create an honest, detailed picture of what life would be like in the fantasy world. Guide their awareness to the possible negative ramifications of each fantasized element by asking reflective questions

such as "Doesn't pain protect us from some things? What are the positive purposes that pain might have? . . . There are advantages to youth, but what are the disadvantages? What are the advantages of age? Are there some gains that come from age which younger people cannot have? . . . Wouldn't eating anything, whenever we wanted, destroy some wonderful eating pleasures that come from anticipating a special food and finally eating it? Wouldn't the foods we really enjoy become less likable if they were all we ever ate? . . . Would it really be an enjoyable state never to experience any changes?"

4. Then, ask them to focus again on their life as it is. Are you speaking to a grandmother? Has she enjoyed time spent with a grandchild? What if her age had frozen at some early stage? What would she not have experienced in life? Once you begin to look at how life would change when subjected to the condition of a fantasy, as in the film classic *It's a Wonderful Life*, most will realize that their lives have brought them much pleasure and be encouraged to enjoy those joys all the more even in the face of illness at the end of life.

THE EXISTENTIAL TRUTH

Existential philosophers realize that sometimes the truth can be cold and harsh, but that fact does not eliminate the possibility of freedom—the freedom not to be victims of that coldness and harshness. From the existentialist's viewpoint, we can choose whether to be victimized by reality or not. We can choose to be the victim of truth or not. The following meditation, called "the Gestalt prayer,"[4] is meant to move people away from being victimized by truth. It is a good meditation for both caregivers and care receivers.

> *I do my thing, and you do your thing,*
> *I am not in this world to live up to your*
> *   expectations,*
> *And you are not in this world to live up to mine.*
> *You are you, and I am I,*
> *And if, by chance, we find each other, it is*
> *   beautiful.*
> *If not, it can't be helped.*

This prayer might at first seem discouraging, but further meditation upon it can bring about a sense of better self-esteem, freedom, and empowerment. Truth also can seem harsh and cold at first, but upon further exploration, it provides moments of solace and growth.

Chiang Tzu's Meditation on Death

The following meditation can offer some comfort in a struggle with truth.

> **Companions**[5]
> *Life is the companion of death. Death is the begin-ning of life. Who understands their workings? Man's life is a coming together of breath. If it comes*
>
> *continued*

> *together, there is life. If it scatters, there is death.*
> *And if life and death are companions to each other,*
> *then what is there for us to be anxious about?*

This meditation, like the previous one, is intended to sug-gest opportunities—in the midst of cold, harsh truths—to enjoy the freedom to respond to truth without becoming its victim.

CHAPTER FOUR

The Right to Be Comfortable

Most of us exercise the right to be comfortable every day. If we are tired of sitting down, we get up, stretch, move around or lie down. If we are bored with staying home, we go out. If we are depressed, we try something that will cheer us. If we feel bombarded with unpleasant thoughts, we divert our attention in another direction. When we are healthy and have choices, these are normal ways of exercising our right to physical and mental comfort.

But when we are unhealthy, our choices to escape pain, boredom, depression, fatigue, or intrusive, unpleasant thoughts are limited. If we become extremely unhealthy, we often do not even have the option of moving our bodies into a more comfortable position. If we are trapped in a terribly uncomfortable position, we don't even have the choice of avoiding unpleasant thoughts. We feel mentally attacked from all directions.

Whenever caregivers can offer some comfort to people facing the end of their lives, we help them meet a profound need. The key to fulfilling this need is giving choices—as many as possible—and honoring the choices that are made.

Russell

Russell, who suffered from lung cancer, had his own diet that consisted of oatmeal, covered with a stick of melted butter, three times a day. This was literally his comfort food. Russell was convinced that this diet helped his body to function at its best during his illness. No one could convince him otherwise.

This diet was Russell's way of making himself feel comfortable. As far as he was concerned, it worked because it kept his energy level high and his bowels regular. That was all he needed, he believed, to be comfortable and content.

What right do we caregivers have to propose an alternate regimen for Russell? Doesn't he have a right to know what makes him comfortable and a right to exercise whatever means he sees fit to achieve comfort?

Andy

A 36-year-old man with AIDS, total blindness, an esophageal ulcer, and HIV cardiomyopathy, Andy was receiving a great deal of pain medication: duragesic patches, nitroglycerine tablets, propoxyphere napsylate tablets, morphine sulfate liquid, and lidocaine viscous liquid.

In the early stages of his illness, Andy adjusted fairly well. He had a strong support from family and friends and an active sense of humor. As his ailments progressed and his physical pain became worse, his medications increased. But after a few weeks of such heavy medication, Andy decided to decrease their intake. He sought an acupuncturist to treat the pain of his peripheral neuropathy, a pain that caused an intense burning sensation. He found acupuncture helpful and was able to discontinue the duragesic patches.

Even though acupuncture was less convenient and gave about the same measure of pain relief as the patches, Andy chose to stay with the acupuncture because, he explained, it was something he was doing for himself, independent of the usual medical directives he received from his caregivers. Because he chose this pain treatment, rather than having it chosen for him, Andy felt empowered. And he felt a certain sense of comfort in simply being able to have the right to determine an aspect of his pain control regimen.

Elmer

Elmer was on morphine concentrate liquid and hydromorphene hydrochloride suppositories for pain because he was dying from lung cancer with celiac disease. The morphine upset Elmer and his wife because they equated it with "giving in" to the disease. To both of them, it meant the disease was out of control, and therefore Elmer's fate was out of their control.

Elmer had never been someone to "give in" to anything. He had been active and self-sufficient for all his 76 years. He needed to have some sense of control over his destiny, some sense that the disease was not victimizing him. He needed to hang on to some control, even if it were only the knowledge that he was doing something for himself.

Elmer felt continual dull aches in his chest. He and his wife decided to treat the aches with reflexology, a therapeutic foot massage. He found the results "very helpful" in relieving his suffering. His wife administered the foot massage, and his morphine dosage was somewhat reduced.

It would be difficult to pinpoint exactly what helped relieve Elmer's pain. Perhaps it was the morphine (though reduced), the loving touch of his wife's hands, the reflexology itself, or a combination of all factors. The important point is not the actual mechanism but the fact that his pain relief was supplemented in a positive way by Elmer's sense of having some choices and control in his fate. This sense was bolstered by his belief that he had a right to feel comfortable, and he had every right to determine how that comfort might be found.

Russell, Andy, and Elmer represent people seeking comfort as a relief from physical stress and pain. But many psychological variables contribute to achieving their comfort. The most important contributor is the sense of having some choice and control. Russell, Andy, and Elmer had the right to be comfortable; they wanted to exercise that right; and they achieved it by choosing comfortable means as each saw fit.

Donald

I met Donald when he was 38 years old and suffering from a brain tumor. His doctor said he had two to four months to live. Except for occasional periods of confusion and mild pain, Donald's mind functioned well. He lived with Liz, his 32-year-old wife, and their two young children. Liz was in the seventh month of a difficult pregnancy.

Donald's doctor had contacted me and introduced me to him as someone who was familiar with brain tumors and had a strong religious background, which was very important to Donald. We became friends quickly over the next two months.

Donald and Liz believed that his brain tumor would soon go away because they had faith in God's healing powers, they lived a moral life, and they were praying that the tumor would disappear. As Donald's pain and confusion increased, he and Liz felt that it was not the tumor's growth that caused these developments, but they were the results of the tumor's being broken up and destroyed by God's healing forces.

As one of Donald's caregivers, I fully accepted Donald and Liz's choice of faith that he would get better. I never talked about his illness unless he raised the subject. I never once implied that anything would happen to him other than what he expected. When he and Liz talked about Donald's saving money for the expected third child's college education, I joined in the conversation with no hint that this notion was impossible.

Donald died three days after his third child was born. Donald had been able to be present at the birth. He and Liz experienced an immense joy that filled his last three days.

Not everyone would agree with the way Donald and Liz dealt with the reality of his illness. Not everyone would approve of my role in supporting their approach. But I cannot imagine a better way for them to handle their situation. It was the best way for them because it was their way. Other people might choose to spend their last two months facing death in what they would call a "responsible" way by rationally exploring all the implications of a man's dying and leaving a young wife and three children. Others might believe that it would be more "practical" to acknowledge that no faith or positive thinking could postpone certain death from a fast-growing brain tumor. Still other people might choose what they would call a "therapeutic" approach of trying to squeeze out every possible benefit that can come from anticipating grief and preparing for the inevitable.

Donald and Liz did make an "irresponsible," "impractical," and "nontherapeutic" choice that contradicted the physical, medical evidence, the "truth" of the last chapter. And I chose to support and assist them. I witnessed two young children and a wife grieving greatly, but I believe two months of "practical" preparation for death would not have resulted in any less grief.

No, Donald did not get the healing result he and his wife expected, but he did indeed find comfort through his faith. Though he was in great physical pain those last three days of his life, he enjoyed a comfort that transcended his pain. Donald was comfortable in what he believed, in who he was, and in those around him: a devoted wife and three beautiful, healthy children.

From my experience with Donald and many other terminally ill and dying people, I have come to advocate this message: Caregivers need to allow and honor people's choices of coping style, even if their style involves complete denial of what we know to be unmistakable facts. Denial preceding death has been likened to blinking in bright sunlight: we cannot look into the sun without blinking any more than we can face death without some denial. We do not want our lives to end, so we deny that possibility as a way of being fully present for those things that we feel are of most importance in our lives. This helps us maintain comfort, and each of us has a basic right to comfort.

As caregivers, we have a responsibility to support the ways that our loved ones and patients choose to cope with their illnesses and destinies. That control is crucial to their survival as death approaches. We should not see their choices as weaknesses if we disagree with them. We also need to recognize that they probably do not wish to be "rescued" by our beliefs, words, or actions. Our job is not to convert them to our ways, but to help them get in touch with their own strength, confidence, faith, spirituality, or whatever else they choose. Through their own choices, they will enjoy their right to comfort.

Alice

Alice appeared as healthy as an average woman in her late seventies. She was spunky and wiry, but she had severe chronic obstructive pulmonary disease. Her physician predicted that death could arrive at any time, and with little warning.

During one of our early visits, Alice told me her philosophy of life: "I get up every morning. I might feel too tired, or I might fall down, but I get up. It's so important to get up every morning—physically and mentally. No exceptions. You've got to get up."

Her simple but profound philosophy kept Alice comfortable and uncomplaining about her own health. She had many other concerns, but not about herself. She worried about her daughter's health, her daughter-in-law's loneliness, her dog's eating habits, her home health aide's workload. She even inquired about my health. But whenever I asked her about hers, she always replied, "Oh, I'm okay. I'm up, aren't I? All I have to do is get up every morning. And I'm here. I'm up."

I might have responded, "Be realistic, Alice. One of these mornings you're not going to be able to get up. Have you thought about that?" But what good would have come from my challenging her reasoning? What benefit could come from destroying someone else's way of coping or finding comfort?

Alice's philosophy proved very realistic for her. She got up every morning as she said she would. Her approach gave her comfort every day, even on the last day of her life. She died in her sleep.

Tools and techniques for promoting the right to be comfortable

ASSESSING FOR THE PHYSICAL DIMENSIONS OF STRESS

Stress is usually experienced in the form of physical symptoms. When caregivers make assessments of those in their care, it is important to gather information that identifies the physical dimensions of stress. The goal is to help patients and loved ones find ways to relieve stress and establish comfort. The following four-part assessment form can be useful in achieving that goal.

Physical Assessment

1. Where is the stress located? Mark the areas where stress is most felt. If there is more than one site, label each site with the letters A, B, C, D, for the most stress to the least stress, and so forth for use in parts 2, 3, and 4 of this form.

_____ head
_____ neck
_____ back
_____ shoulders
_____ chest
_____ arms
_____ hands
_____ stomach
_____ groin
_____ buttocks
_____ legs
_____ feet
_____ joints
_____ other

2. Describe how the stress feels. Place the corresponding site letters in the blanks that most appropriately describe the feeling.

_____ sharp
_____ dull, aching, or diffuse
_____ radiating or shooting
_____ pressing or tight
_____ burning
_____ pulling
_____ other

3. Describe the intensity of the stress on a scale of 0 to 5, with 5 representing the most intense, in the various sites.

Intensity of stress				
	Site A	*Site B*	*Site C*	*Site D*
At present	___	___	___	___
Highest it gets	___	___	___	___
Lowest it gets	___	___	___	___

4. Measure the frequency of stress by checking one for each site:

Frequency of stress				
	Site A	*Site B*	*Site C*	*Site D*
Occasional	___	___	___	___
Frequent	___	___	___	___
Constant	___	___	___	___

5. Determine the patient's view of the stress:
   - What makes your stress worse?
   - Are there times of day or night when your stress is worse?
   - What has helped in the past to control the physical symptoms of your stress?
   - What does the stress prevent you from doing?

It is important to identify several sites of stress because they are often interrelated. The more we can learn about each site and its possible connection to others, the better we will be able to help reduce or alleviate the stress. If stress in one area can be relieved, the others may also become less intense.

Conversely, when one area is relieved, stress might increase in other areas, so it is important to make this assessment carefully.

I strongly recommend that caregivers never assess for problems without simultaneously recommending some steps that patients and loved ones can take to diminish those problems themselves. It is unfair, perhaps even cruel, to raise their awareness of a problem without showing them that they have an ability to address or relieve it. Nor should we leave them with the impression that we are their personal miracle workers.

MEDITATING STRESS AWAY

This activity capitalizes on the natural relaxation that comes through paying attention to one's own breathing and the power of suggestion. If the person in your care is receptive to the following meditation, you should find a quiet place where there will be no interruptions for at least 10 to 20 minutes. Then guide your care recipient through these steps:

1. Sit in a straight-backed chair, feet flat on the floor. If this is uncomfortable, you could sit in a lounge chair with feet elevated.

2. Rest your hands on your lap with the palms up.

3. Close your eyes lightly.

4. As you exhale each breath, release the tension in each part of your body, starting with your feet and going up to your head, one part of your body with each exhalation or two.

5. When your body is relaxed, focus your thoughts on the word "peace." Imagine the emotional state of

being that comes with being at peace with yourself, at peace with your family, and at peace with the world.

6. Now let go of the word "peace" and just be aware of the feeling connected with the word. If other thoughts enter your mind, just observe those thoughts and let them go. Return to the feelings associated with the word "peace" if you need to refocus.

7. After a few minutes, send these feelings of peace to someone else. Imagine embracing that person with all the feelings of peace. Share your abundance of peace with that person.

8. Take a deep breath. Make a full exhalation of that breath. Take one more deep breath and open your eyes.

After this exercise, caregivers and those in their care could discuss how all of us have the power to relax ourselves by concentrating on our breathing and meditating on relaxing thoughts.

OBJECT MEDITATION

Any object that elicits comfort for the person in your care can be suggested as the focus of a daily meditation. Such objects might include a crucifix, a mandala, a statue of a happy Buddha, a picture of a loved one who has died, a picture of a baby, a family photograph, a painting of a pastoral landscape, a mountain, or a lake.

Suggest that the person in your care concentrate on that object and block out any other thoughts. Whenever other thoughts intrude, urge him to will them away and return to the object at the center of the meditation. A helpful way to will away an intruding thought is to imagine a huge hand pushing it away. The hand completely removes the thought and then disappears itself, leaving only the original object as the meditation's focus.

The Bird Meditation

Suggest that the person in your care close her eyes and imagine swans flying across the sky:

One swan enters your field of vision on the left and flies out of vision on the right. Another swan enters and leaves. Then a third enters and leaves.

Imagine several swans flying across the sky. Now picture a completely blank sky, a peaceful blue.

If another thought or picture enters this peaceful blue sky, imagine it being swept away on the back of a swan, carried out of sight like the previous swans.

Continue to imagine the serenity of that peaceful blue sky.

THE GARDEN OF TRANQUILLITY

Caregivers can lead this experience in person or record it on a cassette tape. As with similar exercises, this is most beneficial if you remind those in your care that its effectiveness comes from their power, the power of their imaginations, a power that lets them establish their own comfort.

Traveling through the Garden of Tranquillity
With eyes closed, pay attention to the process of
breathing that is going on inside your body. Instead
of thinking in terms of you breathing the air, think
in terms of the air breathing you. . . . The air, on its
own accord, is entering your body and then leaving
your body. Entering and leaving. . . . Entering and
leaving. . . . Entering and leaving.

You are making no effort whatsoever. You are
simply allowing the air to come in and go out, come
in and go out. . . . You are making no effort. You
are merely allowing. . . .

Now allow a picture to enter your mind.
A picture of a large garden with red roses every-
where. . . . You are in that garden and you are
walking among those red roses. Your walking is
almost like floating. You are floating through this
large garden of red roses. . . . You breathe in the
deep fragrance of the red roses. . . . These are roses
of life-giving energy. . . . These are roses of joy. . . .
These are roses that bring a comforting smile to
your face. . . .

Find the most beautiful red rose that you can
find. . . . Look at its beauty. Examine closely all
of its beauty. . . . Inhale the fragrance of this red
rose. . . . Examine its intricacies. . . . This red rose
is a symbol of your life energy. It is a symbol of your
passion. A symbol of your enthusiasm. . . . Breathe

in that energy. . . . Breathe in that passion. . . .
Breathe in that enthusiasm.

Up ahead of you, you see the garden of red roses
changing into a garden of violet roses. . . . You walk
and float toward the violet roses, walk and float to
the center of that section of the garden so that all
you see now is violet roses. . . . In the center of
this part of the garden is a large chalice, a chalice
that is emitting a violet flame. . . . The flickering
of this violet flame conveys sanctity. . . . This is a
sacred violet flame. It is the flame of harmony. It is
the flame of cleansing. It is the flame of forgiveness.
. . . All these violet roses carry the same symbolism.
These roses symbolize harmony. They symbolize
cleansing. They symbolize forgiveness. . . .

In the midst of all these violet roses, you feel that
all of this symbolism is directed toward you. You are
in harmony with all that is around you. . . . You
are being cleansed. . . . You are being forgiven. . . .
Feel the forgiveness. . . . Breathe in the fragrance
of forgiveness . . . You are completely forgiven . . .
All people have forgiven you, and you have even
forgiven yourself. . . . You forgive yourself for not
being perfect. . . . You accept yourself for everything
that you are. . . .

Up ahead of you, you see the garden of violet
roses changing into a garden of pink roses. . . .
You walk and float toward the pink roses, walk

continued

and float to the center of that section of the garden so that all you see is pink roses. . . .

In the center of this section of the garden is a beautiful bed of pink rose petals, soft pink rose petals beckoning to be laid upon by you. . . . You walk and float toward that beautiful bed of pink rose petals and lie down upon them. . . . You smell the comforting fragrance. . . . You feel the relaxing softness. . . . You realize that these pink roses symbolize love. . . . You are encircled by love. . . . You smell love. . . . You feel love. . . . Your inner being says, "I know I am loved. . . ." You are loved. . . . You are loved completely. . . .

After resting upon these roses of love, you slowly rise and start walking and floating toward the section of the garden that is filled with white roses. . . . Soon you are completely surrounded by pure white roses. Everywhere you look, there are pure white roses. . . . These are creamy white roses of purity. . . . Here you are surrounded by perfect peace. . . . Here you are surrounded by divine peace. . . . Breathe in the fragrance of peace. . . . Here all your worries and fears are gone. . . . Here is your true home, your home of peace. . . . You are at peace. . . . Everywhere is peace . . . You are at peace.

And now, you are choosing of your own free will to come back to this room. In coming back, you will be returning with everything that you have received in this garden. . . . You are returning, having experienced complete forgiveness. . . .

> *You are returning, knowing that you are fully*
> *loved. . . . You are returning, knowing that you are*
> *at peace, totally at peace. . . . You may now slowly*
> *open your eyes.*[6]

EVOKING COMFORT

The following exercise can be suggested as a way of promoting comfort from anxiety or pain.

1. Guide your care recipient into a relaxed mood by suggesting that he concentrate on his breathing. Ask him to concentrate on the word "comfort" and think about the many ways it could be defined.

2. Ask him the following questions. He could write the answers, or you could do it for him if he is unable.

   - How would you describe your body when it is feeling comfortable?

   - How would you describe your various emotions during times of comfort?

   - What physical surroundings would be most helpful to you in achieving comfort?

   - What types of people make you comfortable?

3. Ask him to think about how much he values times of comfort, how much he desires to have comfort.

4. Ask him to imagine all the physical sensations of comfort, to let all his tension melt away.

5. Suggest that he internally repeat the word "comfort" with each time he exhales breath. This could be done for several minutes.

6. Urge him to stay comfortable throughout the rest of the day, to resolve to be a model of comfort. Suggest that he resolve to emanate comfort.

7. Suggest that he make a large sign with the word "comfort" on it; use colors he finds comforting; place it in a prominent spot where he might often need to feel comfort.

THE RECIPE FOR COMFORT

This recipe for comfort can be used when the person in your care feels stress, anxiety, disturbing thoughts, or some type of physical pain. It can be written on a recipe card and placed in a convenient place to be pulled out whenever needed. The goal is to forget completely whatever is causing the stress, anxiety, or pain by the time all the steps are completed. Like any recipe, no step should be omitted.

Recipe for Relief

1. Name three continents and two countries in each of those continents.

2. Snap your fingers ten times.

3. Recite the alphabet backward.

4. Blink your eyes ten times.

5. Hum the tune of your favorite song.

6. Take twenty deep breaths, counting to yourself with each exhalation.

7. With your eyes closed, try to picture all the details of the setting of your favorite vacation.

A PEACEFUL MEDITATION

Ask the person in your care to close her eyes as you slowly lead her through the following meditation that uses guided imagery.

A PEACEFUL MEDITATION

Get as comfortable as you possibly can. Concentrate on the word "relax." Relax. . . . Relax. . . . Relax. . . .

Concentrate on the word "peace." Peace. . . . Peace. . . . Peace. . . .

Imagine the most peaceful location that you can possibly envision. . . . Imagine a very serene place. . . . What does that place look like? . . . Look in all directions at this peaceful place. . . . Relax in this peaceful place. . . .

Now, still keeping your eyes closed, imagine the most pleasant smell that you can possibly imagine. . . . Imagine breathing in this serene fragrance. . . . Relax as you breathe in this calming fragrance. . . .

Now, imagine the most soothing taste that you can possibly imagine. . . . Imagine savoring this pleasant taste. . . . Relax as you taste peace. . . .

Now, imagine the most relaxing touch that you can possibly imagine. . . . Imagine being caressed and held with this comforting touch, being peacefully caressed and held by someone you love very dearly. . . . Relax as you are gently touched by this loved person. . . .

Relax as you see your peaceful scene. . . . Relax as you smell that soothing fragrance. . . . Relax as you taste that pleasing taste. . . . Relax as you are caressed and held with peaceful touch. . . . Relax. . . . You are at peace. . . . You can relax. . . . Peace. . . . Peace. . . . Peace. . . .

DYING BEFORE DEATH

Several religious traditions suggest that their adherents face death in all its reality before it arrives. Such traditions ask them, in effect, to die emotionally and spiritually before dying physically. The objective is to die to the normal ways of the present world in order to live more fully and transcend the fears of death. Hindus refer to this as *moksha*. Buddhists call it *nirvana*. Practitioners of Zen refer to it as *satori*, Muslims as *fana*, and Christians as "being born again." The premise is that there is a positive, comforting effect that comes with "dying before death."

Caregivers can help their patients and loved ones try to achieve some of these comforting effects by encouraging them to write a dialogue between themselves in the present and themselves after death. The dialogue could include questions or general conversation between the two parties. The longer the dialogue, the better. After it is written (or tape-recorded if that is preferable), the dying person may be willing to share and discuss it with a caregiver.

Some people who have written such dialogues feel they get "a new lease on life," but not everyone has positive results. Caregivers should be prepared to respond appropriately to whatever responses might come forth.

GOD'S BREATH

The more relaxed a person's breathing, the stronger its calming effect. This meditation activity can relax the breathing pattern so that it brings calm to both emotions and body. It is designed for people who have a somewhat traditional religious background. But it can be appropriate and helpful to others if it is preceded by a dialogue about its content.

The words are from the first and third verses of a popular Christian hymn.

> *God's Breath*
> *Breathe on me, Breath of God, fill me with life anew, that I may love what Thou dost love, and do what Thou wouldst do.*
>
> *Breathe on me, Breath of God, till I am wholly thine, till all this earthly part of me glows with Thy fire divine.*

Explain to the person in your care what will happen in this activity, and share the words that will be used for meditation. Ask her to concentrate on her breathing, making the breaths fuller and deeper. Eyes may be open or closed, whichever is more relaxing.

Suggest that she feel more and more relaxed as she inhales and exhales each breath. As you encourage her to relax, match your own breathing pattern with hers, so that the two of you are inhaling and exhaling at the same time, as though you both share the same lungs. Continue encouraging relaxation and matching your breathing pattern with hers.

Keeping the same breathing pattern, softly verbalize a phrase from the hymn with each exhalation, as she meditates on your words:

1. First exhalation: "Breathe on me, Breath of God."
2. Next exhalation: "Fill me with life anew."

3. Next exhalation: "That I may love what Thou dost love."

4. Next exhalation: "And do what Thou wouldst do."

5. Next exhalation: "Breathe on me, Breath of God."

6. Next exhalation: "Till I am wholly Thine."

7. Next exhalation: "Till all this earthly part of me."

8. Next exhalation: "Glows with Thy fire divine."

Repeat the meditation three, four, or five times. After several repetitions, softly say the word, "Relax," every third exhalation until you have the sense that she is truly relaxed.

BUDDHIST MEDITATION

For comfort, someone who is approaching the end of life might want to meditate daily upon the following quotation.

> *To die artfully is to die thinking of nothing, wishing for nothing, wanting to understand nothing, clinging to nothing. . . . Just fading away like clouds in the sky."*[7]

The following exercises and activities, through the end of this chapter, are intended for caregivers' use in reducing our own stress. If we can become more relaxed, we will be better able to increase the well-being of our loved ones and patients.

ASSESSING OUR INTERPERSONAL STRESSORS

To help ourselves and our care recipients, we would do well to relieve our own stress. If we can be more relaxed, we will not only feel better, but those in our care will absorb our comfort rather than our stress. But in order to provide the most comfortable atmosphere for our loved ones and patients, we need to sort through our own stressors. This activity can begin the process.

1. Under each of the following headings, write the names of people who cause you some stress in each category:

Supervisors and authority figures	Business associates and fellow workers	Family, friends, and other acquaintances
————	————	————
————	————	————
————	————	————
————	————	————

2. Place check marks by each name to rank the amount of stress in your relationship with that person. Use one check mark to denote some stress; two check marks when stress is usually as present as it is absent; three check marks when stress is almost always present, with few if any periods of no stress.

3. Reflect on these two questions:
   - What common characteristics do people with two and three check marks have?
   - What are all the various emotions you feel when you think about these people? Name those emotions.

4. From these reflections, determine particular types of people or situations that you need to avoid. Are there certain areas where you could work on decreasing stress with these people and situations? A combination of these two solutions might be ideal.

MANAGING STRESS AWAY

Caregivers often experience stress because we don't have enough time to do what we feel we need or want to do. Improved time management can help us alleviate our own stress and if possible, the stress that we pass along to those in our care. Here are some tips for better time management and less stress:

1. List your goals; what are your goals for your personal life? for your job? for your community?

2. Label one third of those goals as high priority, one third as medium priority, and the final third as low priority.

3. Work on the high priority goals first.

4. Work on medium priority goals next, when time allows.

5. Eliminate, postpone, or delegate low priority goals.

6. Use your creativity to try to accomplish two or three goals with one task.

7. Use your creativity to figure out ways to accomplish some aspects of your goals during normally wasted periods of time (standing in the checkout line, waiting in doctors' offices, riding to work).

8. Set time limits for accomplishing each goal. Eliminate any goal—or temporarily put it on hold—if it is not accomplished during the set period of time.

Periodically repeat the above process to see if your goals continue to have the same values and priorities.

MANAGED STRESS REDUCTION

Another way for caregivers to manage stress away is through planning. Like previous activities, this one reduces our stress so we can pass on more comfort to our patients and loved ones. Here's the plan:

1. Make a list of specific activities that frequently lead to feelings of stress.

2. Identify just one of these activities and concentrate on it.

3. Work on reducing the stress of this activity by the following process outlined in this "Stress Reduction Planning Sheet." Examples are suggested in parentheses.

Stress Reduction Planning Sheet

1. Activity producing stress (A professional caregiver becoming too attached to someone in her care):

2. What I can do about it (She could establish a relationship with a counselor):

3. A major obstacle to doing that (She might worry about not knowing how to find a good counselor):

4. What I could be doing (She could ask people to recommend counselors whom they know):

5. What I will do (She gets references, chooses a counselor, makes an appointment, and starts counseling before the end of next month):

6. My goal (She would commit to five sessions):

7. My reward for accomplishing my goal (She could buy herself a new pair of shoes):

8. The results that I expect (Satisfactory resolution of the previous problems and a plan to prevent similar problems in the future):

9. Evaluation of results (A self-administered test for anxiety or stress would be done before counseling, at the end of counseling sessions, and two months after counseling ends).

RELAXING BREATHING FOR CAREGIVERS

Find a quiet place where you will not be interrupted for the next 10 to 20 minutes. Sit in a straight-backed chair with both feet placed flat on the floor.

Rest your hands on your lap with your palms up.

Lightly close your eyes.

Draw your attention to your natural breathing pattern. Notice the complete route of the air as it fully enters your body and fully leaves your body. Do this for a couple of minutes.

Inhale a large amount of air through your nose. Hold it for a few seconds. Then exhale through your mouth. Practice this breathing method for a couple of minutes.

Return to your natural breathing pattern. With each inhalation, feel the naturally peaceful relaxation that comes into your body. With each exhalation, feel all your stress leaving your body. Do this for a couple of minutes.

Rest in that state of peaceful relaxation. Realize that it takes no effort whatsoever to breathe. Just rest.

IMAGINING STRESS AWAY

This guided imagery could be read to you by a coworker or friend, or tape-recorded. Remember, if it works for you, you may want to use it with those in your care.

YOUR SPECIAL PLACE

While in a comfortable position, close your eyes and center your attention on your feelings. . . . Sense the particular feelings that you have when I say the following words, "peace, . . . " "contentment, . . . " "freedom, . . . " and "safety. . . . " Now, with those feelings in your consciousness, imagine a place that you know, a place you remember, or a place that is completely imaginary. Imagine that place characterized by peace, contentment, freedom, and safety. Whatever place comes into your consciousness, stay there in your mind. . . . Do not let other places or thoughts intrude. If they do, keep returning to that place of peace, . . . contentment, . . . freedom, . . . and safety.

continued

Become completely absorbed in this place. . . . Imagine the soothing feelings that permeate your entire body. . . . Imagine the relaxing sounds that you hear in this place of peace. . . . Try to sense the soothing aromas that are present in this place. . . . Examine what is around you. . . . Examine what is below you. . . . Examine what you see in the distance. . . . Examine what is close to you. . . . Examine everything that is contributing to your peace, ... contentment, . . . freedom, . . . and safety.

This is your special place. . . . This place belongs completely to you, and you may come here whenever you want. . . . Whenever you are anxious, you may close your eyes and go to this place of peace, . . . contentment, . . . freedom, . . . and safety. . . . This is your special place. . . . Once again, examine this place with all of your senses: the sights, . . . the sounds, . . . the aromas. . . .

You are about to leave this place. But you may return whenever you wish. All you need to do is just close your eyes and travel in your imagination. . . . For now, say good-bye to the soothing aromas. . . . For now, say good-bye to all the pleasant sights. . . . For now, say good-bye to the peace, . . . contentment, . . . freedom, . . . and safety. . . . Whenever you are ready, knowing that you can always return, slowly open your eyes. . . .

MEDITATIONS FOR A CALM CENTEREDNESS

Caregivers can use either of the following meditations to find a calm centeredness that can be fostered in themselves and those in their care:

When we label some deaths right,
*   other deaths become wrong.*
When we label some deaths good,
*   other deaths become bad.*
Living and dying create each other.
The easy way and the difficult way are
*   interdependent.*
The long life and the short life are relative.
The first days and the last days accompany each other.
Therefore, the true caregiver of the dying does all
*   that needs to be done without asserting herself,*
*   and says all that needs to be said without saying*
*   anything.*
Things happen, and she allows them to happen.
Things fail to happen, and she allows them to fail
*   to happen.*
She is always there, but it is as though she is not there.
She realizes that she does nothing,
*   yet all that needs to be done is done.*

In letting go,
*   there is a gain.*
In giving up,
*   there is advancement.*

Do not practice controlling.
Practice allowing.

continued

> *Such is the mystery of happiness.*
> *Such is the mystery of wealth.*
> *Such is the mystery of power.*
> *Such is the mystery of living and dying.*

THE CAREGIVER'S CONTINUAL REMINDER

When things do not turn out as we would wish, the psychotherapist Albert Ellis offers advice that he calls the "elegant solution."[7] This solution is found in accepting the fact that it is not the end of the world if the worst possible things happen. If our patient or loved one is continually angry at us, it does not mean we are the most terrible caregivers. If someone in our care dies in excruciating pain, we are not the most awful, unworthy caregivers. None of us is perfect. None of us cares for a perfect person. No one is unworthy of life when things go terribly wrong. Each of us has tomorrow. Each of us has some redeeming value. The world goes on, so we try harder, try something else, or simply accept the fact that there is nothing else that can be done. And we are not terrible caregivers if that is the case.

RESPECTING THE CARE RECIPIENT

One of the best ways to provide comfort is to offer respect. We naturally feel comfort when we know that we are surrounded by people who respect us for who we are and how we behave, people who respect our philosophies and our coping styles. As caregivers, we need to respect patients and loved ones, whether we agree or disagree with them.

CHAPTER FIVE

The Right to Touch and Be Touched

Most of us take for granted a baby's need to be touched. When we see an infant, we cuddle it, stroke its head, touch its soft arms and legs, let it wrap its tiny fingers around our finger. We recognize that children need touch to understand that they are loved, to feel secure, and to learn trust.

Many people overlook older people's desire for touch. Yet recent studies have shown that the need for touch increases with age and during times of stress and social isolation. As one woman said, "I want my last sensation to be someone holding my hand." Caregivers of elderly people who are experiencing stress and isolation would do well to recognize touch as an integral part of our caregiving skills.

Anna

The memory is more than 15 years old, but still crystal clear. As Anna lay in bed, she appeared comatose, unresponsive, with the heavy, labored breathing that often closely precedes death. She was alone in the room when I entered. I felt uncomfortable, awkward. I wanted to stay just a moment. I had only promised her family that I would stop by and say a prayer at her bedside. I thought that I'd quickly do my duty and move on to someone else, someone more conscious of my presence.

Anna's skin was very white and etched with years of wrinkles. She had a terrible aroma. I was aware of her breathing, the labored breathing of nearby death. Her pale, lifeless left arm was dangling over the side of her bed. I thought it would be more decent to lift it and place it alongside her body before I began the prayer, so I gently reached for her hand. I jumped with a start. Her hand squeezed mine violently and held it in a grip that turned my knuckles white. Yet her comatose appearance remained the same in every other way.

I was unable to move. I felt embarrassment rushing to my face and sweat beading on my forehead. Her grip froze me—my feet felt nailed to the floor. I couldn't leave the room without dragging her with me. There was no way I could ignore her. I was forced to look at her.

Though pale and deeply wrinkled, Anna had a beauty about her, a deep beauty. Great character was written on her face. I began to notice little details: her gentle lips, her flowing hair, her smooth forehead. I tried to imagine the color of her eyes. I wondered, What does her voice sound like? What was her favorite music? Did she enjoy her life? What would her smile have looked like?

Her grip remained tight, but I began to lose all my uncomfortable feelings. I realized that I had a ridiculous grin on my face. Unexpectedly, tears filled my eyes as I thought: I had almost totally disregarded this woman. I had almost treated her as if she were not a human being but an inanimate object. Tears kept coming. I couldn't stop them. I was crying uncontrollably.

Anna suddenly drew a great breath of air into her lungs. I saw her smile. She let go of my hand. She died.

I stood there, still crying. What had happened? Who was she? How much time had passed? I sat down on the floor and cried more tears, sad tears, happy tears, plain tears.

In recalling that memory, I am overcome with the awareness that everything that happened centered around the power of touch. Both Anna and I needed to be touched so very much. Anna wanted touch. She needed touch. She had a right to touch and be touched.

Tools and techniques for promoting the right to touch and be touched

The desire to exercise the right to touch and be touched can be a strong one, but it is not universal. Part of recognizing this right is respecting someone's choice about when touch is inappropriate—when it may be the wrong time, the wrong dose, or the wrong person. We honor the person and that right when we let him decide if he wants to touch or be touched.

FOOT WASHING

You will need a comfortable chair, a large basin of warm water, some pleasantly scented soap, soft washcloth, soft towel, and skin lotion or oil. With your patient or loved one in a comfortable chair, soak her feet in the warm water for several minutes. Slowly cleanse her feet with the soap, warm water, and washcloth. Pat her feet dry with the towel. With the skin lotion or oil on your palms, caress and massage her feet. You may want to repeat the washing to remove the lotion or oil, though some may not need to be washed away. Afterward, put soft slippers or socks on your care receiver's feet to keep them warm and well moisturized.

SENSUAL BACK RUB

First create a sensual, relaxing environment. A quiet time in the evening might be best. Ideally, the room should be slightly warmer than normal. Soft music could be playing in the background. The room might be lit only by candles—scented candles for added ambiance. The phone could be unplugged.

The care recipient should lie facedown on the bed with no clothing on the back. Gently, slowly clean the back with a damp, warm, soft washcloth. Pat it dry with a soft towel. Gently rub body oil onto the back until the entire back has a thin coating. Your hands might need to be immersed in oil again periodically and rubbed together as you apply enough oil to cover the back completely.

Awaken the back's sensory capacity by patting it with your palms or gently chopping with the edge of your hands. Tap all over the back with your fingertips. Use one or two fingers and your thumbs as if they are legs walking up and down and all around the back.

Stroke, rub, and knead the back. Imagine that you are sending loving energy from the center of your being out through your fingertips. This step would involve the most amount of time of all the steps.

Again, tap all over the back with your fingertips. With a thumb or index finger, print messages of caring on the back. Ask her to guess what you are writing. Sample messages: "We have had some good times together." "You are so beautiful." "I care so much for you." "You are such a good wife (husband, father, mother, partner, or friend)."

Finally, gently and slowly clean the back again with a slightly damp, warm, soft washcloth and pat it dry with a soft towel.

Nourishing Touch

In discussing the right to be in control in chapter 1, we saw how an occasional alteration in our normal conversation—a change in choice of words, phrases, questions—can enhance caregivers' relationships with people in their care. The same is true with touch. By changing our normal patterns of touch, we can bring a new sense of connectedness and intimacy to these relationships.

If your typical greeting or farewell is a three-second handshake with cursory eye contact, try lengthening the handshake ten seconds and making direct eye contact. Or you might hold the hand without shaking it, or grasp the hand with both of yours, or follow the handshake with a quick hug.

If your normal greeting or farewell is a firm bear hug, try softening it, or place your hands on the person's shoulders as you give a gentle massage. You might ask to receive a hug rather than always initiating one yourself, or you might substitute a kiss on the cheek.

By altering your usual greeting or farewell, you force yourself to think about what you are doing. This brings more sincerity to gestures that often become routine. The receiver of your new greeting or farewell will feel your sincerity, and a new sense of connectedness can flourish between you.

HUG CARD

For some people, particularly those who have difficulty expressing themselves, a "hug card" is a useful prop. Caregivers could give them a card on which "Please give me a hug" is printed. Simply offering them the card does not necessarily mean that they have to use it, but it is there as a resource if they choose to use it.

THE LAYING ON OF HANDS

When someone is near death, this activity involves the entire circle of family and friends. They stand around the bed, touch the dying person, and say words of comfort. One at a time they say special messages that they wish to convey through their touch. For example, relatives and friends touch her head, hands, feet, shoulders, arms, and each person might say:

> Grandmother, I am sending you all my love through my hands. . . .
>
> Grandma, I am sending you all my happy memories of our times together as I hold your hand. I am remembering all the times you came to our house with a special surprise hidden behind your back, and all the special warm hugs you gave me. . . .

Mother, I am remembering all the times I came running home from school, crying. You would hold me with your gentle arms until I stopped crying. I am sending all that love back to you through my hands.

Thank you.

For caregivers to promote others' rights to touch and be touched, we need to maintain and occasionally revitalize our own physical natures. When we are about to begin any activity involving touch with patients and loved ones, for example, it is important that we be as stress free as possible. If we bring our own tension to exercises, we may very well pass it on to them. The following three activities can help us become more relaxed before we start our work and can also help us carry on that work more effectively.

TOUCH WITHOUT TENSION

This meditative imagery activity can be led by a fellow caregiver or friends, or can be listened to on tape to help ease our tensions and prevent us from passing them on.

> *Find as comfortable a position as you can. . . .*
> *Remove eyeglasses, loosen any constrictive clothing. . . .*
> *Close your eyes. Focus on how comfortable your*
> *body feels. . . . Feel how your comfort increases as*
> *you take deeper breaths. . . . Feel the tension expel*
> *from your body with every exhalation. . . . As you*
> *continued*

*breath deeply, you are breathing out tension, . . .
uneasiness, . . . and stress.*

*As you breath out tension, feel the muscles in
your body relaxing more and more. . . . You feel
your chest muscles relaxing. . . . You feel your facial
muscles relaxing. . . . You feel your neck muscles
relaxing. . . . You feel your back muscles relaxing. . . .
You are exhaling all of your troubles. . . . You are
exhaling all of your tension. . . . You are exhaling
all of your uneasiness. You are exhaling all of your
stress. . . .*

*Your lungs are one of the most efficient elimina-
tors of waste you have in your body. Let your lungs
work for you. Let your lungs take away all of
your tension. . . . Let your lungs take away all
of your uneasiness. . . . Let your lungs take away
all of your stress. You are relaxed. . . . You are at
peace. . . .*

*Remember that your comforting lungs are with
you wherever you go. So whenever you feel stress,
remember that you can always just close your eyes,
sense your breathing, and fully relax. . . . In a few
minutes, you will be slowly opening your eyes.
However, remember that you can always return to
this state of relaxation. In the future, all you will
need to do is just close your eyes, breathe deeply,
and let the natural calming effect of your breathing
provide you with this wonderful, peaceful healing. . . . You may now slowly open your eyes. . . .*

GETTING IN TOUCH WITH TOUCH

Because caregivers serve people in the final phase of life, we continually need to keep sensitizing ourselves to the value of our own physical nature and the value of touch. Here are five suggestions to help us maintain that sensitivity.

- Have a regular physical exercise routine.
- Be conscious of how we treat our bodies through what we eat.
- Be conscious of how we treat our bodies through our grooming habits.
- Practice touching and hugging in as many settings as possible.
- Receive occasional massages from professionals.

BODY REVITALIZATION

This is another exercise that can help us revitalize ourselves, strengthen our inherent powers, and rest ourselves.

- Get in a relaxing mode by doing some deep, focused breathing.
- With your eyes closed, picture your whole body and identify places that feel dull, . . . places that feel alive, . . . places that feel pain.
- Direct your focus toward the part of your body that is most in need of positive energy. This part of you could be in pain, aching, tense, or just tired. Imagine

moving the sensations felt in the "alive" places to the places of pain, fatigue, and dullness.

- While focusing, choose a color that you associate most with vitality. Imagine that color permeating that part of your body with invigorating energy.

- Feel that part of your body become stronger with each inhalation of breath. Feel strength with each inhalation, and feel relaxation with each exhalation.

CHAPTER SIX

The Right to Laughter

Most people feel somber, uncomfortable, or awkward when they approach someone nearing the end of life. They check the fun-loving side of their personalities at the door. They don't consciously intend to deprive an elderly or dying person of humor or the lighter side of life, but that is exactly what happens. Laughter may be rippling from the next room or down the hallway, but too often an older or dying person is cheated by the excessive seriousness of many visitors and caregivers. Why do we assume that someone nearing death doesn't want to laugh and hear others laugh?

Several recent studies reveal that laughter is desired even as the end of life approaches. In one survey that offered a choice between seriousness and humor, 83.6 percent of people close to death chose humor.[8] Another research study found that 85 percent of terminally ill patients felt that humor would be helpful in their care, yet only 14 percent said they actually experienced humor from their caregivers.[9] And another researcher concluded that "so much valuable ordinariness, richness, and warmth are lost because of the false solemnity which [people] feel from others. They begin to feel excluded from the ordinary human realm."[10] In other words, when we don somber masks, we place a barrier between our humanity and theirs. Humor is an essential reminder of the joys of being human.

Harry

Harry had multiple sclerosis. When he contracted pneumonia, he landed in the hospital. But Harry wasn't one to enjoy confined spaces like a cramped hospital room. He wanted to "walk" whenever possible: from his bed to a chair, to the bathroom, or just to exercise a bit. But Harry's preferred, and sometimes requisite, style of "walking" took the form of Harry needing one person to hold him around the waist from behind while Harry held the waist of someone else in front of him—a shuffling kind of three-person train with an engine in the front and a caboose at the rear while Harry, the freight, went along for the ride.

Struck by the humor of this silly-looking but often necessary formation, Harry would loudly and often repeat, "Chug-chug-chug-chug-chug-chug-chug-chug-choooo-woooooo!" Whoever was playing engine or caboose at the time always broke into giggles.

One morning, Harry decided to alter his routine when he needed to go to the bathroom. Two female nurses answered his buzzer, automatically fell into position, one in front, one in back, and expected his usual train noises. After a minute or so of silence, Harry suddenly jerked forward, then jerked backward, and said, "La Cucaracha." This triggered a laugh from the surprised nurse behind Harry, and it spread to the front nurse and then Harry himself. As they chuckled, Harry's surgical pants slipped to the floor. This ratcheted up their laughter until all three were laughing so uncontrollably that they collapsed to the floor. Now their raucous uproar began attracting staff and visitors to Harry's door. After ten or fifteen minutes, the laughter ran its course, but people who experienced Harry's train story still get good feelings when recalling it several years after his death. Harry continued to share his joke and his right to laughter well after his death.

Humor is essential in everyone's life, but it may be even more so during the terminal phase of an illness. When someone nears the end of life, the prospect of death is confusing for everyone involved. But humor can help us detach, step back for a moment, and see this prospect with more objectivity. A good laugh can restore perspective and momentarily reduce frustration, anxiety, and even panic. When a situation seems unbearable, such as having to have two nurses accompany you to the bathroom, humor can offer strength and help us focus on whatever seems too overwhelming to bear.

By laughing in the face of death, we grasp a measure of control over the seemingly uncontrollable. In laughing at our own weaknesses and infirmities, we assert a power over them. Such laughter is a means of defense and control, fragile though it is.

As important as humor is, caregivers should remember that it is not always fitting or appreciated. Not all terminally ill people will find humor appropriate. Just as with touch, we first need to assess the appropriateness of humor before launching into a joke or a humorous story. One way to predetermine whether it will be welcomed or suitable is to use this guideline: Appropriate humor becomes inappropriate when it is offered at the wrong time, in the wrong dose, or to the wrong person.

That is a general statement, but you can apply it to each person and individual situation. Look for signs, feel your way along, until you can fairly accurately predict the individual's reaction to the humor you are about to inject. If you sense that humor is desired, you can lighten the moment with a funny comment or story. Whenever appropriate—but only when appropriate—the opportunity to laugh is a great benefit to the people in your care.

Tools and techniques for promoting the right to laughter

THE SIGNS OF STRESS RELIEF

People who are dying have sometimes said that they experience fear in the eyes of others. So if you wear a solemn face when you enter the living space of someone in your care, you will most likely get stressful results. Instead of that expression, try to replace it with one that conveys more lighthearted feelings. The following suggested "Stress Relieving Signs" can be placed in patients' living areas to signal visitors that they might leave their feelings of fear and solemnity outside.

THIS IS A FROWN-FREE ZONE.

DANGER: EXCESSIVE SERIOUSNESS CAN PROVE HAZARDOUS TO YOUR HEALTH.

NO BUSINESS TRANSACTED HERE EXCEPT FOR FUNNY BUSINESS.

I COULD DIE LAUGHING IF YOU WOULD BE WILLING TO TELL ME A JOKE.

I AM NOT AFRAID OF DEATH. I JUST DON'T WANT TO BE THERE WHEN IT HAPPENS.

EVERYONE ALLOWS JOY TO COME IN THIS ROOM: SOME
WHEN THEY ARRIVE, SOME WHEN THEY LEAVE.

A FUNNY OPERATION

The following imagery experience capitalizes on some images that might be particularly funny for someone in the
final phases of life. Discussion centered on perceptions, feelings, and thoughts could occur afterward.

DR. LAUGHALOT OPERATES

Close your eyes. . . . You are about ready to have a
very unusual operation, one that is different from any
operation you have ever had or ever heard about. . . .
Dr. Laughalot will be the chief surgeon. . . . In this operation, all of your serious bones are going to be removed and replaced with funny bones. . . . In this operation, all the heaviness in your heart and head will be
removed so that you are very light hearted and light-
headed. . . . Unfortunately, you could not afford a complete facelift as part of this operation—and your insur-
ance won't cover that. . . . But you will receive a partial
facelift at both corners of your mouth. . . . Finally 124
tickle implants will be placed throughout your body. . .
. Take some time to imagine what kinds of effects this
complete operation would have on you. . . . Imagine
how you would behave after this operation. . . .

How would you interact with your family after
this operation? . . . How would you interact with your

continued

friends? . . . How would you interact with your professional caregivers? . . . How would people perceive you after this operation? . . . What kinds of effects would you have on them? . . . What feelings do you have after this operation? . . . Picture yourself at a shopping mall. How would you behave at that shopping mall? . . . Picture yourself at a library. How would you behave at that library . . . Picture yourself at somebody's funeral. How would you behave while attending a funeral? . . . After this operation, what three words would you use to describe yourself?

Now go back to how you were before the operation. How did you interact with other people before you had this operation? . . . How did people perceive you before this operation? . . . What kinds of effects did you have on them? . . . Before the operation, how did you behave when you went to the shopping mall? . . . How did you behave at the library? . . . At funerals? . . . In three words, how would you have described yourself before the operation?

Think about what traits you had before the operation that you would like to keep with you always. . . . Think about what traits you had after the operation that you would like to keep. . . . Realize that you have all these traits inside yourself right now. . . . What traits do you want to bring out more? . . . What traits do you want to bring out less? . . . As we are ending this experience, I would like you to open your eyes slowly. . . .

FUNNY VIDEOS

Video stores are stocked with humorous videotapes, new and old. Think of some of your favorites, or take recommendations from your patients, or ask the store clerks or your movie-going friends for some particularly funny ones. When people are ill or limited in their mobility, they and their caregivers can watch these tapes together. The experience is even more fun if you can share popcorn, ice cream, or candy.

A FUNNY LIFE REVIEW

The following activity uses the principle of recalling a past event and reliving it in the present to bring more humor into the present situation. Caregivers would ask those in their care to choose three questions from the following list. Suggest that they not answer them right away, but save their answers for your next visit. Giving them some time to respond will not only assure a good time for the next visit, but it will also provide them with some light moments in between visits.

Ten Funny Things to Ponder

- What do you remember as a funny thing that happened to you in grade school?
- What is the funniest thing that ever happened to you during a meal?
- What is the funniest thing that ever happened to you when you were not fully clothed?
- What is the funniest thing that ever happened to you in an automobile?

- When did you injure yourself and cause you or someone else to laugh?
- What is the funniest joke that you have ever heard?
- What is the funniest joke that you have ever heard that has religious subject matter?
- What is the funniest thing that you have ever seen a child do?
- What is the funniest thing that you have ever seen an older person do?
- What is the funniest thing that you have ever seen on television?

Short Imagery Experiences

The following imagery exercises can promote laughter. They also could help to put caregivers and those in their care on a common level, the level of vulnerability. Begin these "vice versa" experiences after asking the person in your care to close her eyes.

Vice Versa

Visualize your doctor standing in front of you. . . . Visualize your doctor sitting down in front of you. . . . Visualize your doctor sitting on a toilet. . . .

Visualize your nurse giving you a shot. . . . Visualize yourself giving the nurse a shot. . . .

Visualize a member of the clergy preaching to you from the pulpit. . . . Now visualize yourself in the pulpit, preaching to a congregation of clergy. . . .

WHAT STRESS?

The following exercises can help caregivers relieve some of their own stress with a few laughs and reinvigorate themselves so that they can facilitate some humor for those in their care.

If caregivers are under stress, we cannot meet the urgent needs of the people in our care. And we are hardly in the mood to bring humor to them. This activity can divert us from our own stressful state:

Pull out the following list of activities whenever stress seems overpowering. Complete each activity in the order listed as fast as you can. If you reach the end of the list and still feel stressed, repeat the list in reverse order.

Raise your eyebrows twenty times.

Shout five words that begin with the letter "z."

Rub your tummy ten times counterclockwise and ten times clockwise.

Swallow five times.

Roar like a lion. Bark like a dog. Purr like a kitten.

Clap your hands ten times.

Throw something up in the air and catch it—twelve times.

Stick your tongue out five times.

Make five different silly faces.

Shout five words that begin with the letter "q."

LAUGHING FOR DOLLARS

Caregivers can reward ourselves for helping people in our care to laugh. For each time in a day that you get the laugh from your patient or loved one, give yourself an award of a dollar credit. Three laughs, three bucks at the end of the day. At the end of the week, tally your credits and treat yourself to whatever you'd like, a meal, a book, a compact disc, an item of clothing.

THE CAREGIVER'S FACIAL MAKEOVER

To bring laughter to those in our care, we need to signal a readiness for humor. We communicate this largely by our facial expression. This exercise can help send those signals:

Every time you see your face in a mirror, look for signs of tension: a furrowed brow, narrowed eyes, clenched teeth, tight lips, jutting chin, scrunched neck.

When you notice these signs of tension, initiate a conversation with that tension. Gently persuade your face to loosen up.

After your face has relaxed, deliberately tense it up again. Then relax it. Tighten it up again. Relax once more. Alternate this tightening and relaxing for a couple minutes.

When you have finished this alternating routine, practice making a relaxed, gentle smile.

MORNING MEDITATION

A Zen Buddhist practice recommends going directly to a mirror immediately upon waking and making ridiculous postures and facial expressions. Try it. Laugh the whole time, or at least smile the broadest of smiles. Laughing at ourselves in the mirror is easier for some of us than for others, especially in the morning. Try this exercise first thing each morning for about two or three minutes.

CHAPTER SEVEN

The Right to Cry and Express Anger

Many caregivers discourage people in the last phases of their lives from crying or being angry. Perhaps we are uncomfortable around sadness and anger, so we attempt to smooth over others' distress. We may think we are helping someone near death by trying to erase or ignore these emotions when we say, "Don't cry. . . . Oh, cheer up. Things will get better. . . . Don't upset yourself. . . . Don't waste your time and energy on anger. . . ."

Some caregivers even label anger and tears as "immature," inferior ways of coping with the many trials and tribulations that inevitably accompany the last phases of life. Yet all of us need outlets for expressing a wide range of emotions— regardless of our age or state of health. As physical pains and frustrations increase toward the end of life, the need for outlets certainly increases. Even if caregivers see these emotions as "negative," we need to respect the fact that they need to be expressed. People nearing death have a right to express those emotions.

If caregivers try to squelch anxiety, immense sadness, anger, fear, and similar feelings, we add to our patients' and loved ones' already heavy burden of facing death. We should be attempting to ease, rather than add to, their burdens. We should not restrict their expressions of emotion, or try to re-direct them, or gloss over them—even when those emotions are difficult for us to witness. If we want to allow them to die with dignity, we need to allow them to die in their own way, and that way may include tears and anger.

Susan

I could not understand what made Susan so easygoing. If I were in her position, I would probably be weeping a great deal, and I would have been extremely angry. Cancer was eating away at her face. Her life was being taken away while she was in her late forties. The physical ravages of her disease kept her from going anywhere in public. And she would never be completely free of pain until she died.

Susan certainly had much reason to be angry and sad, yet she was so serene—almost cheery—with everyone. I asked her once, when I was visiting her at home, "What's your secret, Susan, for staying so calm in the midst of all that is happening to you?"

"Follow me," she replied. "I'll show you my secret."

She led me to a spare bedroom, opened the door, and said that this was her "release room," a room where she would go when-ever she felt hurt, angry, or very sad. When she needed to release some of these emotions, she entered this room to cry or express anger. The room was simply furnished with a bed, one chair, and two large stuffed animals, a bear and a giraffe.

When she needed to cry, Susan explained, she would lie on the bed, hold the stuffed bear tightly to her, and sob until she felt completely cried out. When she was angry, she would either sit on the chair and yell at the giraffe (toward which she projected some identity, such as her disease or a person who had been unkind), or she would wring the giraffe's long neck with all her strength.

Her "release room" helped her immensely, Susan told me. By providing her with an avenue to vent her emotions, it allowed her to be calm and easygoing with me and other caregivers and in situations that would normally cause great anger and frustration.

Anger may seem "negative" to some people, but it has its place even in the last phases of life. It can provide an experience of power at a time when so much of a dying person's former powers have been sapped or stolen. Anger can give a sense of being in charge of one's own life and death, and it can stave off the fear of the isolation of dying.

Crying also has its benefits. As everyone who has cried his or her "heart out" knows, it drains away emotional toxins and clears the mind and body so that we can regain our strength. For people nearing death, the right to cry and express anger offers an opportunity to feel power and potency, which renews their energy for the physical and emotional trials that lie ahead.

Tools and techniques for promoting the right to cry and express anger

Anger Time

Caregivers can encourage friends and relatives of care recipients to give them a daily, regularly scheduled "anger time."

During this 15- to 20-minute period, the patient or loved one should be left alone completely. Move out of hearing range. Encourage them to shout, throw or pound things—whatever they wish to do to express their anger.

HITTING, RIPPING, AND STOMPING ANGER AWAY

Caregivers can suggest the following activities to help those in our care vent their anger:

- Lie facedown on a mattress and pound your fists into the mattress as you yell and scream. Do this until you are completely exhausted or until you break into tears. Let the tears flow.

- Roll up a newspaper or magazine and hit it against a bedpost or door frame, as you shout the name of a person or thing that is the focus of your anger. Do this until you are completely exhausted or until you break into tears. Let the tears flow.

- Find a newspaper or old telephone book, a crayon or marking pen. Write in bold letters a word that comes to mind about your anger. Say the word with feeling. Rip the piece of paper to shreds. Then stomp on it. Keep doing this until you run out of paper, words, or energy.

- Find someone who is willing to have a pillow fight. Project all the causes of your anger onto this other person. Have a pillow fight until you either start crying, or laughing, or expend all your energy.

THE IMAGINARY SLEDGEHAMMER

Suggest to the person in your care that she imagine all the restraints that have ever been placed on her since childhood until the present. These restraints would be anything that has kept her from becoming whatever she wanted to become or prevented her from doing whatever she wanted to do. (Some examples might be an interrupted education, family responsibility, financial limitations, or illness.)

Suggest that she imagine these restraints one at a time, take an imaginary sledgehammer, and destroy each and every restraint until it is totally smashed in her imagination.

RELEASING ANGER

Not everyone is willing or accustomed to expressing anger openly. This exercise can help people who have difficulty expressing strong, negative emotions.

Caregivers can suggest that the person in their care close his eyes and picture an imaginary chalkboard and chalk. Ask him to write about his anger on this chalkboard. Urge him to use the most graphic language he can, including words he might be embarrassed to say aloud. Suggest that he write furiously, imagining strong and bold strokes of the chalk. In this way, his anger is expressed both in what is said and in how it is "written." Now suggest that he stand back, in his imagination, and look at the chalkboard. He should read and reread what he has written. Finally, ask him to take an imaginary eraser and furiously erase everything on the chalkboard.

Here: Try Me

If caregivers are willing, you might offer to be the target of your patient or loved one's anger. This can help someone who is experiencing a great amount of anger.

Offer yourself as the recipient of verbal anger. Allow the person in your care to create a role-playing situation in which you play the person or thing that is causing his anger. Let him verbally dump all over you.

You might also offer to be the recipient of physical anger by suggesting that he release his anger by squeezing one of your arms or legs as hard as he can. Again, you would play the role of the person or thing that is causing his anger. You could encourage him verbally by saying, "Squeeze harder. Get it all out."

It Is Okay to Cry

Many people have reasons to cry, but for whatever personal reasons, they don't. They may feel embarrassed to cry, or see crying as a sign of weakness. They may have wanted to cry for a long time but have not found a time or opportunity when they felt it was fitting or comfortable to shed their tears. This short, simple exercise is intended for them: Every once in a while, caregivers should remind them that it is okay to cry, that they need to give themselves permission to cry, that it is always all right to give ourselves permission to cry.

Oh, Tractor!

If the person in your care is in a setting where swearing would be considered inappropriate, suggest that he use creative alternatives to common swear words. When the urge to cuss hits, he would have two or three words to summon from his new "swearing" vocabulary—whatever words he chooses like "Tractor! . . . Fudge! . . . Sugar! . . . Cork! . . ." These have sounds that can be pronounced with feeling. He can spit them out with all his might without offending anyone who might be within earshot.

The last seven exercises were for patients and loved ones, but caregivers also become angry, frustrated, and sad on occasion. We need to be careful in expressing our own anger because it could be potentially destructive for those in our care if they are already emotionally fragile. As we have discussed elsewhere in these pages, we need to manage our stress regularly in order to be effective caregivers. That doesn't mean that we should smother or hide our feelings, but if we monitor our own stress regularly, we will be better able to understand its causes and to discover how we can relieve that stress. When we are able to manage our stress, we let ourselves be open for the sadness and anger of those people in our care, and we allow them maximum accessibility to the right to cry and express anger.

ONGOING MONITORING OF THE CAREGIVER

The following "stress log" can help caregivers monitor stress in an ongoing manner; several copies of this sheet could be made for this task. I have structured this format with three columns, each for an individual stressful event, but you may want to make several more columns if that fits your needs better.

Stress Log			
	Event 1	*Event 2*	*Event 3*
Date/time of day	_____	_____	_____
Cause of stress	_____	_____	_____
Physical and emotional reaction to the stress	_____	_____	_____
Intensity of reaction (on a 1–10 scale with 10 as highest)	_____	_____	_____
Method used to relieve the stress	_____	_____	_____
Intensity of stress after method (on a 1–10 scale)	_____	_____	_____
What was learned about stress and stress relief	_____	_____	_____

CHAPTER EIGHT

The Right to Explore the Spiritual

A few years ago, a colleague named Michael Maher and I conducted a survey of terminally ill patients and discovered that most have a strong desire to talk about religious or spiritual issues—even people who said that they had not been involved with organized religion of any kind. Over 50 percent of people without previous religious involvement said they wanted to discuss spiritual issues. We also found that this desire increased markedly as death became imminent. Other researchers have reported similar findings.

We caregivers need to respect the right of people in the final phases of life to explore religious and spiritual issues. We can honor that right in two ways: by providing an atmosphere for them to talk freely about such issues and feelings, and by not imposing our own beliefs or thoughts on them.

When we enter a relationship of spiritual exploration with an open, receptive attitude, we discover a truly vast realm of spirituality. The longer I am involved with hospice work and its philosophy of receptivity toward others, the broader my perception of spirituality becomes. I have found that spirituality can indeed come in a wide variety of packages. At times, it may be very mystical and enigmatic, as the following stories demonstrate. As caregivers, we need to be open to experiences that we can neither label nor define. We must be ready to encounter anyone's spirituality, which can be totally other and ungraspable to us.

Hazel

When I first met Hazel, I was informed that her doctors expected her to live no longer than two months. Hazel didn't concur. She intended to extend her prognosis, and she did—another nine months.

During that time, Hazel had a profound influence on many people around her, including me. Although her brain tumor prevented her from speaking more than one- or two-word sentences at a time, Hazel was the center of interaction wherever she went. She had a special way of spontaneously evoking conversation in others.

Over the last five months of her life, she insisted on attending her church almost every Sunday. Even though she had to attend services on a gurney, and she could not hide the disturbingly obvious physical effects of her disease and therapy treatments, Hazel was always busily engaged in conversation. Her contribution to any conversation was not with words but with watchful, knowing expressions. Her eyes communicated total involvement. Her face conveyed the impression that she always knew more than anyone else. Everyone who knew Hazel felt that she was in touch with a reality greater than the physically obvious. We sensed that she was somehow attuned to a spiritual reality.

My last visit with Hazel was evidence of both her uncanny ability to evoke a conversation through her facial expressions and her spiritual dimension. I entered her room at the nursing home and pulled up a chair by her bed. As I reached out and held her hand, I relayed the well-wishing of various friends and acquaintances. Hazel's watchful, knowing eyes were turned toward me the whole time that I spoke. After about five minutes, I stopped chatting and simply held her hand as I looked around her room. I noticed the television set, greeting cards, flowers, the institutional beige walls. When I turned back toward Hazel, her eyes were still trained on me. I gave her a little smile and resumed glancing around her room silently, but I felt that her eyes were definitely saying something to me, something about the room itself.

"This room is kind of silly, isn't it? A really silly space," I blurted, puzzled by my own words.

Hazel's expression did not physically change, but I felt that it was saying she was in agreement with my words. I nodded with a half smile. Her gaze continued. A few minutes of silent reflection slipped by as I continued to hold her hand. I looked into her eyes again and added, "My words are kind of silly, too, aren't they? Words are kind of silly."

Her eyes were still locked on my face. I felt my thoughts confirmed. With a grin, I again reflected in silence, my eyes slightly downcast. When I looked up once more, I said, "And I am kind of silly, too. I'm very silly. We're all very silly people, aren't we?"

I waited a few moments, looked into Hazel's eyes again, and said good-bye with a big, foolish grin.

After leaving her, I got in my car and drove around. What had I done? Was I crazy? Had I done anything other than make a complete fool of myself? I wondered as I drove aimlessly. I felt embarrassed and frustrated. Yet I also sensed something else as I recalled Hazel's eyes. I perceived something was going on inside her that was far beyond my comprehension. It seemed that she was in touch with something very powerful, spiritual—something that was flowing from her watchful, knowing eyes.

At the end of Hazel's funeral service a week later, the minister asked all two hundred people in attendance to rise and give Hazel a standing ovation. An unusual occurrence, certainly, but no one hesitated. Everyone stood and applauded for several minutes. Many people beamed smiles, others sobbed, and some wore dumbfounded looks.

What had happened? I wondered. Was everyone crazy? What was going on? Were people projecting spirituality onto Hazel? Or was she transporting spirituality into others?

Jack

After Jack retired as a vaudeville magician, he opened a mail-order business selling magic tricks. I had known him for several years when his wife asked me to visit him quickly. Doctors expected Jack to live only another 24 hours. She warned me that he had a high temperature, was hallucinating, talking nonsense, and did not recognize her.

As I stood in the doorway of his hospital room, I saw Jack propped upright in bed, surrounded by pillows. He smiled and said, "Doug, we have all been waiting for you to arrive."

I wondered who "we" were because he was the only person in the room. I walked in, smiled at him, and thought that this might not be such a difficult visit after all.

"Today is your initiation day, Doug. Today you will become a member of the Royal Society of Magicians," Jack said.

This is going to be a fun visit, I thought, and I wanted to participate in his fun.

But Jack then looked away from me, and his expression seemed glassy-eyed. He spoke several nonsensical sentences that sounded like both a magical incantation and a "speaking in tongues." Then I realized that I had always sensed that Jack approached magic as if it were a religion.

He abruptly broke off his nonsensical language and looked directly at me. "Come closer," he said in a serious tone.

"You will learn a great magic trick today, the very greatest trick of all." His voice was weak but determined. "Come closer."

I felt that I was already near enough to see or hear whatever he was about to do or say, but I leaned in, over his bed.

"Come closer," he repeated.

I began to feel uncomfortable, but I leaned in until we were eye to eye with not more than six inches between our faces. Jack seemed to be looking straight through me. His eyes were searching for something in my eyes.

Without any change in his facial expression, Jack whispered, "Watch me disappear."

His eyes took on a glassy, frozen appearance. I knew instantly that Jack died in the moment he whispered those words.

A huge wave of feelings rushed over me: shock, wonder, sadness, warmth, coldness, oneness, hollowness, confusion, peace. I knew that Jack had invited me to share in a most powerful event, an event of his own design and making.

I have related Jack's story not simply because it is dramatic but also because it shows how one man can exercise his right to be in control of his dying process. For Jack, this was a magical, spiritual choice. For me, it was an incredibly positive experience, a mysteriously enriching event with profound spiritual undertones.

But let's look at this experience from another angle: What if I had walked into Jack's room and contradicted him with logic? "What do you mean 'we', Jack? There's nobody in this room but you"? What if I had urged him to quit talking "nonsense" and face reality? What if I had tried to rein in his "hallucinations" with reasoned arguments instead of letting him set his own agenda? I would have been making some terrible mistakes if I had tried to impose my notions on him.

Jack wanted to die in his own unique way. He had chosen to be a magician in life, and he wanted to die a magician. So Jack chose the best possible death he could imagine for a magician. Throughout his adult life, he exercised his right to be in control and his right to have his beliefs respected. In his last hour, he continued to exercise those rights. And I am grateful that he could do so with respect and appreciation.

Jim

On my first meeting with Jim, his wife, Barbara, greeted me at the door of their home. She whispered, "Jim is having a rough day. Please don't stay too long. He's very tired."

As the three of us sat around their kitchen table and chatted, I sensed that Jim wanted me to stay, and Barbara couldn't wait for me to leave. Jim was wearing a tie, dress shirt, sharply pressed slacks, a vest, jacket, and a wig. He was animated and showed no sign of fatigue. Barbara, in a plain housedress and apron, looked quite tired. I decided to compromise between their expectations and stay about half the usual time for an initial visit. In that brief span, I did not have enough time to assess Jim's spirituality, which I would normally do as part of a general assessment. I left hurriedly and forgot my overcoat.

Later that day, Jim telephoned. Could I come by at five o'clock and pick up my coat? I asked whether I could drop by somewhat earlier, but he insisted on five o'clock specifically.

I arrived exactly at five. Jim greeted me at the door. No longer wearing his wig and now in blue jeans, he said warmly, "Come in and sit down. Would you like anything to drink?"

I knew Jim was ready to talk because he quickly mentioned that Barbara was in the basement, under a hair dryer, and would probably be down there for another forty minutes.

"Mind if I have a beer?" he asked.

"No," I replied, as he opened the refrigerator. Jim opened the beer can, sat down across the table from me, and plunged into conversation.

"You know what I miss most? I miss going down and having a beer at Stormy's Bar. Stormy ran that place like a church, at least the way a church ought to be run."

"Bingo!" I thought. We are about to discuss spirituality.

Jim proceeded to tell me how Stormy's Bar operated as he thought a church should be run: no betting, no swearing, no fighting allowed. Stormy didn't serve anything but beer. Yet certain vices were permitted. Stormy's patrons could swig their beer, smoke, and tell jokes as long as there was no swearing in the jokes.

According to Jim, that was the way a church should be run. A church needs some rules, he thought. A church needs to acknowledge that there are some things people should not do. Yet it should also acknowledge that nobody is perfect. Everybody needs a little leeway. The church should recognize that everyone has a few vices, vices that are just part of being normal. Such a "religion" would mean people could relax in knowing that they were fully accepted as they were, in spite of occasional vices.

For Jim, such a church would also proclaim that people did not have to impress others by their mannerisms or clothes—just as any attire was permissible at Stormy's Bar. And, like Stormy's, a church should have an open atmosphere where people can say whatever they like. They didn't have to say anything unless they believe it. They did not have to say that they agree with others if they really did not agree. Jim believed that the same freedom of expression that existed at Stormy's should prevail in church as well.

Like Stormy's Bar, a church ought to allow people to be unique, natural, and fully accepted in spite of occasional disagreements and minor vices, as long as they didn't infringe on others' dignity, Jim believed. For him that was spirituality. That was religion. That was Stormy's Bar.

David

The first symptoms were only a shortness of breath and an unrelenting cough. But when David's physician discovered a whitish coating on his tongue, he suspected that David might have AIDS. The diagnosis was soon confirmed, and David's problems grew. Meningitis developed. His weight dropped from 170 to 130 pounds in just a few months. The AIDS progressed rapidly. Confusion and memory problems quickly became evident.

As David was being consumed physically by his disease, he was simultaneously being consumed by a religious searching. Whenever he was able, he read the Bible. When reading became too taxing or he could no longer hold the Bible, he asked others to read it to him. He begged readers not to stop reading until he fell asleep. If a reader stopped too soon, David's eyes would open and his facial expression sent a clear message: "Keep reading until I am asleep."

He also watched and listened to religious programs on television and radio. He wanted these left on even while someone was reading to him and after he fell asleep. David would not tolerate any other programming. He could not get enough religious input. He was on a religious quest, one from which he would not be diverted, one that permitted no interference under any circumstances. That was his choice.

People in the last phases of life have the right to be accepted—totally accepted—for who they are. This applies particularly to their spiritual beliefs and choices. We have no business imposing our beliefs or thoughts. Our job as caregivers, family members, and friends is not to convert, preach, evangelize, or "reason with them" in any way, whether overtly, covertly, obviously, or ever-so-subtly.

Instead, we caregivers should practice just the opposite. We should be as receptive as possible and respect their spiritual beliefs and preferences. If we are believers ourselves, and they are not, we must respect their lack of belief. Our task is to support the people in our care by giving them our presence, by being with them in complete, unconditional acceptance. If we do this, we can help them find and use their own emotional and spiritual strengths.

Tools and techniques for promoting the right to explore the spiritual

A Spiritual Assessment

The following questions are carefully worded so as not to impose any belief system. Those questions that use theological language are phrased to address important issues without confronting or offending the people in our care.

1. When you want to feel strength, where do you go, who do you see?

2. When you want to feel comfort, where do you go, who do you see?

3. In one sentence, how would you describe the purpose of your life?

4. What one goal do you have that is most important to you right now?

5. How would you respond if someone asked you, "Do you believe in God?"

6. How would you respond if someone asked you, "Are you ready for your life to come to an end?"

7. Do you believe in any kind of existence after this life?

Asking someone directly, "Do you believe in God?" can be confrontational and offensive. But asking, "How would you respond if someone asked you, 'Do you believe in God?'" is not. Yet both questions probe the same information.

THE JOURNEY ANALOGY

By our choices of religious vocabulary, we may reveal our own religious preferences and possibly offend others. We may not intend to impose our beliefs, but careless word choices can bring that inadvertent result. Some examples: referring to the "Old Testament" in the presence of Jewish people; mentioning the phrases "being born again" or "sacraments" to some Christian people; assuming Judeo-Christian perspectives with people who are not of Judeo-Christian heritage.

As you use the following metaphoric conversations with people in your care, keep in mind the possible pitfalls of religious vocabulary. After these conversations, two follow-up scenarios are provided as examples.

LIFE IS A JOURNEY

Sometimes people use the analogy that life is a journey. If you were to describe your time now as coming toward the end of a journey, how would you describe this last portion? For example, a walk across a desert? . . . a climb up a mountain? . . . an ocean voyage?

What one thing do you feel you most need to do before your journey is over? . . . To what extent do you sense a power greater than yourself present with you on this journey? . . . What kinds of thoughts and beliefs are you having at this time in your life's journey? . . . What worries you the most at this time? . . . What helps you feel relaxed and peaceful at this time in your life? . . . Whom do you most want to be close to you during this

continued

time? . . . What do you want most from that person? . . . What can I personally do for you while you are on this journey?

EXAMPLES OF FOLLOW-UP SCENARIOS

_____, you have just described your journey as a walk through a desert. Do you prefer the desert experience? . . . Would you like some kind of refreshing oasis in the middle of the desert? . . . If you would like to find an oasis, what would it be like? . . . . How might I help you create that oasis? . . . .

_____, I see that the end of your journey is very terrifying to you. Is there another possibility for the end of your journey? . . . . If you were to imagine the best possible end to your journey, what would it be like? . . . . How might we together explore that as a possibility? . . . .

THE SACRED SHRINE

Caregivers can present the following suggestion as an avenue to spiritual exploration if the people in our care seem willing to discuss it.

> Many people believe in powerful forces beyond what can be seen or touched. Some people believe in a personal Higher Power, some in a Christian God, some in a Hindu God, some in a Divine Force that is inside everyone, some in a Divine Nature, some in Divine Energy.

There are many names and descriptions of how people perceive such powerful forces. I would like to learn about how you view what many people label as Divine. Between now and my next visit, I would like you to construct a "Sacred Shrine" that expresses what you feel about a power that is greater than yourself. Choose some place in your home, a bookshelf, an end table, dresser top—wherever you want to build this shrine. Put various items that somehow symbolize your concept of a force, or forces, greater than yourself. Those items might be pictures, mementos, special objects, certain books. When I come back next time, I would like you to explain to me what is at your Sacred Shrine.

PICTURING THE DIVINE

Another suggestion for a caregiver to initiate spiritual exploration:

People have different impressions of the Divine. Some think of it as a creative force, some as an angry person, some as a loving person. Some people do not believe that the universe has a Divine aspect at all.

I invite you to draw your impressions of the Divine, if you have any impressions. Draw the Divine however you see it. Try to be very creative. Draw a picture that differs from a picture you have ever drawn, a picture that captures all your feelings and thoughts about what is Divine. If you do not have a concept of the Divine, draw a creative picture that expresses your feelings when you are around people who talk about the Divine.

THE SPIRITUAL JOURNAL

Caregivers can encourage patients and loved ones to keep a written journal that records their daily thoughts about God, afterlife, religion, or anything else that is related to spirituality. Each entry would be labeled with the date, time, and occasion. People in our care should be given the opportunity to share some of the entries with us if they choose.

A LETTER FROM YOUR HIGHER SELF

For anyone who has a strong concept of what is sometimes called "a god within," this ten-part activity can help to explore that thought more fully:

1. Ask him to focus on his breathing, feeling the air bring comfort to his entire body.

2. After focusing on that comfort, ask him to find a place in his body where the greatest amount of comfort is felt; ask him to direct his full consciousness to that part of his body.

3. Suggest that he imagine shifting that sensation of comfort to another part of his body where comfort is needed. Tell him to let that comfort permeate his entire body; let that comfort fill every pore.

4. Ask him to concentrate on his feelings; he may find that other thoughts arise. Ask him to notice which feelings are associated with discomfort and which ones are associated with comfort.

5. Suggest that he can make choices about where to direct his consciousness. Draw attention to the immense power that we all have through our ability to choose the direction of our consciousness.

6. Ask him to transcend his thought processes and to take a wider, deeper viewpoint. Suggest that he imagine that he actually chose to be born, that he imagine that he lovingly chose to possess this body, these feelings, and this mind.

7. Urge him to accept fully the volition involved in becoming who he is today, to examine fully all the major choices involved in creating this body, these feelings, and this mind. Remind him that there was a concern for self and a love of self that was behind all of these personal choices.

8. Ask him, "What message of love do you wish to say to this person who is you? What loving message do you want to say to the person that you have chosen to be?" Urge him to write these thoughts in the form of a letter to himself.

9. Suggest that he put the letter in an envelope, seal it, and address it to himself.

10. Suggest that he give the letter to a friend to hold until a time arrives when the friend feels that the letter might be most needed.

SPIRITUAL AFFIRMATIONS

In the last phase of life, an individual may want two or three of the following affirmations placed nearby as reminders to internalize their meanings. The word "God" is used in these affirmations, but the person in your care may wish to substitute another, such as "Jesus," "Spirit," "My Creator," "Allah," "Yahweh," "The Energy of the Universe," or "All of Creation."

> I will soon be held in the arms of God.
>
> God's love has been made just for me.
>
> I am getting closer and closer to God.
>
> God and I are soul partners.
>
> Soon there will be no difference between me and God.
>
> Make room for me, God. I am coming.
>
> This is a day that God has made. I will rejoice and be glad in it.
>
> I am closer to God in pain than in pleasure.
>
> Although I walk in the shadow of death, I will not be afraid since God is with me.

PALMS TOGETHER, PALMS UP

This activity can be used by anyone who has a sense of a spiritual presence or a desire for a spiritual presence. Again, other words can be substituted for the word "God."

1. Ask your patient or loved one to put her palms together as a symbol of a desire to turn over concerns to a higher power.

2. She may then pray something like, "God, I give you my worries about my declining health. I release to you my fears of dying. I surrender to you all my anxieties about these upcoming weeks."

3. Suggest that she concentrate on giving up her worries and releasing her fears.

4. Then ask her to turn her palms up as a symbol of her desire to receive from this higher power.

5. She may then pray something like, "God, allow me to receive your love, your patience, your calm centeredness, your guidance, and your joy."

6. Ask her to conclude this activity with ten minutes of silence during which she would reflect on this process.

DEDICATING THE PROCESS

Whatever hardships people experience in the last stages of life, they can use those hardships as a means of dedication to God. This activity can help them achieve that.

1. If they are in pain, they can pray or meditate on an example such as this: "I dedicate this pain for the sake of God. Through this pain, I am reminded of the impermanence of that which is human, so that I might turn to an everlasting God. Through this pain, I am being drawn into a readiness for that everlasting God."

2. If they can no longer be allowed complete nourishment, they might pray or meditate: "I am fasting for the sake of God. Through this fasting, I am reminded of the weakness inherent in being human, so that

I might turn to an omnipotent God. Through this fasting, I am being drawn into readiness for the omnipotent God."

3. If they are feeling very lonely, they can pray or meditate: "I am experiencing loneliness for the sake of God. Through this loneliness, I am reminded of the smallness of humanity, so that I might turn to the omnipresence of God. Through my loneliness, I am being drawn into a readiness for that omnipresence of God."

INSPIRATION THROUGH EXPIRATION

Invite the person in your care to spend a few minutes concentrating on the breathing process in order to achieve a feeling of natural relief from tension.

Suggest that he pray inwardly as he breathes; for example, "I exhale my anxiety. I inhale God's peace. I exhale my loneliness. I inhale God's presence. I exhale my pain. I inhale God's comfort."

Ask him again to concentrate on his breathing pattern, while reflecting on the previous prayer once more.

A HOLY CONVERSATION

A caregiver would lead the following imagery experience by reading it aloud. Although the text uses the name "Jesus," it can be varied appropriately. A person of the Jewish faith might have this imaginary conversation about death and afterlife with Moses. A Buddhist might imagine talking with the Buddha, while a Muslim might converse with Mohammed.

CONVERSATION WITH JESUS

Close your eyes and imagine that you are being transported to Gethsemane. . . . You see Jesus all alone, kneeling and praying. . . . You can see his power. You can also see his vulnerability. You see all of his internal struggles. . . . You quietly walk over to his side and kneel next to him. You kneel there in silence. . . . After a short while, Jesus turns to you with love in his eyes and asks, "What can I do for you?" You look Jesus in the eyes and say, "Please tell me how you feel as you are facing death. . . ." Imagine how Jesus responds to your request while he is in Gethsemane. . . .

Now imagine that you are being transported to the foot of Jesus' cross. . . . You see Jesus hanging alone on that cross. He is in great pain. He feels completely deserted. . . . After a little while, Jesus sees you standing below him. With love in his eyes, he asks, "What can I do for you?" You look Jesus in the eyes and say, "Please tell me how you feel as you are facing death. . . ." Imagine how Jesus responds to your request as he is hanging on the cross.

Now imagine that you are being transported to the throne of the resurrected Jesus. You see Jesus relieved of all his pain, basking in the glory of God. . . . You quietly approach his throne. You kneel in silence. . . . After a little while, Jesus turns to you with love in his eyes and asks, "What can I do for you. . . ?" You look Jesus in the eyes and say, "Please tell me how you feel after you have died. . . ."

continued

> Imagine how Jesus responds to your request after he has experienced the resurrection. . . .

After this imaginary conversation concludes, the person in your care may want to discuss it further with you. Be ready to listen, but don't push it.

I Am Holy

Here is another guided imagery experience that caregivers can lead to promote the right to spiritual exploration.

Discovering Our Holiness

Close your eyes and imagine that you are walking across a vast desert. The desert is hot. . . . The desert is dry. . . . The desert is barren and lonely. . . .

You are lost, without any direction, without any purpose. You feel discontented. You feel uncomfortable. You are alone, without friend or companion.

You realize that there have been many times in your life when you have experienced similar feelings. You realize that there have been many moments when your life felt just like this hot, dry, lonely desert. . . . Perhaps you are now in one of those times when you feel very little purpose, very little contentment, very little companionship. . . .

Be aware of these feelings as you imagine yourself walking across this desert. You see the hot sun. . . . You see the dry sand. . . . You see the empty horizon. . . . As you are looking at that lonely horizon, you see some gathering clouds way off in the distance. . . . Mighty, billowing, glorious clouds. The clouds are also gentle and powerful. You know that they are being sent by a loving God. . . . As the clouds come closer, you grow more aware that they are God-given clouds, intended just for you. . . . Clouds that are being sent to bring you rain, rain that will wash away all your troubles. . . .

These mighty, billowing clouds are now directly over your head, blocking the hot rays of the sun. . . . From the clouds, a gentle, cleansing rain falls. . . . You turn your face to the sky and feel the raindrops wash your face. . . . This rain washes away all your shortcomings. Every shortcoming that you have ever had is being washed away by this gentle rain. . . . All of your mistakes are being washed away. Every mistake you have ever made is being washed away by this gentle rain.

As the rain continues to fall, you look around and see that the desert is gradually turning into a luxuriant garden. . . . Trees are sprouting up before your eyes. They are reaching for the sky. . . . Green grass is growing out of the sand, creating a lush carpet as far as you can see. . . . Flowers, red, yellow, pink, are blossoming around the tree trunks and blooming throughout the green grass. . . .

As the rain gradually stops, you feel the rainwater slowly evaporate from your skin. . . . The clouds are drifting away and revealing a new sun, a pleasantly warm, welcoming sun. A relaxing sun. A God-given sun. . . .

continued

You see a rainbow in the sky. . . . You hear birds singing.
. . . You see butterflies fluttering among the flowers. . . .

As you breathe in the fresh air, the God-given air,
you feel all your burdens being taken away. . . . As you
breathe in the fresh, God-given air, you feel your body
straightening, you chin rising. You feel proud of who
you are. . . . You feel loved just as you are. . . . You feel
content just as you are. . . .

The pleasant warmth of the sun cradles you. The fresh
air permeates your body with its freshness. . . . You are
encircled with warmth. You are saturated in freshness. . . .
You are encircled with love. . . . You are saturated with
love. . . . You are encircled with contentment. . . . You
are saturated with contentment. . . . You are at peace. . . .
God is fully with you. God will never leave you. . . .

THE INDWELLING GOD-ESSENCE

This meditation could be used by caregivers as well as those
in their care.

*I am a point of light within the mind of God. I
am a point of love within the heart of God. I am
a point of manifestation within the body of God.
I am a point of creativity within the activity of
God. I am a point of awareness within the great
enlightenment of God.*[11]

A Meditative Prayer

This well-known prayer of St. Francis of Assisi offers an opportunity for rich meditation. It does not have to be confined to the Christian tradition.

> *Lord, make me the instrument of your peace. . . .*
> *where there is hatred, let me sow love;*
> *where there is injury, pardon;*
> *where there is doubt, faith;*
> *where there is despair, hope;*
> *where there is darkness, light;*
> *and where there is sadness, joy.*
>
> *O Divine Master, grant that I may not*
> *so much seek to be consoled as to console;*
> *to be understood as to understand;*
> *to be loved as to love;*
> *for it is in giving that we receive;*
> *it is in pardoning that we are pardoned;*
> *and it is in dying*
> *that we are born to eternal life.*

Inward–Outward–Inward Prayer

Caregivers could lead those in the later stages of life through the following prayer, which both acknowledges the negatives and positives within each of us and brings the positives to the forefront.

With eyes closed and hands over your eyes, concentrate inwardly. . . . Say to yourself, "There are parts of me that are weak. I have weakness. . . ." Say to yourself, "There are parts of me that are lonely. I have loneliness. . . ." Say to yourself, "There are parts of me that are afraid. I have fear. . . ."

Keeping your eyes closed, take your hands off your eyes and place them in a posture of receiving, palms up. Concentrate. . . . Say to yourself, "I am capable of receiving strength. I am asking for that strength. . . ." Say to yourself, "I am capable of receiving love. I am asking for that love. . . ." Say to yourself, "I am capable of receiving comfort and peace. I am asking for that comfort and peace. . . ."

With your eyes still closed, return your hand to cover your eyes. Concentrate. . . . Say to yourself, "There is strength within me. I have strength. . . ." Say to yourself, "There is love within me. I have love. . . ." Say to yourself, "There is comfort and peace within me. I have comfort and peace. . . ."

With your eyes still closed and your hands covering your eyes, rest. . . . Say to yourself, "Rest, knowing that I have strength. . . ." Say to yourself, "Rest, knowing that I have love. . . ." Say to yourself, "Rest, knowing that I have comfort and peace. . . ."

Whenever you are ready, slowly take your hand away from your eyes and slowly open your eyes. . . .

Last Words

This exercise may not be appropriate or comfortable for everyone, so a caregiver should consider it carefully before initiating it. If you decide to use this exercise with an individual patient or relative near death, it can prompt a beneficial discussion at its conclusion.

Suggest to the person in your care that he imagine himself out walking on a sunny day. As he is walking, he sees a soccer ball roll into the street. A little boy runs out after the ball just as a car enters the street going well over the speed limit. To protect the boy, the care receiver lunges forward, pushes the boy out of the way, and gets hit by the car himself. People rush out and gather around him. As he is lying there, he realizes that he will only live a couple more minutes. With his final breath, he looks up to the gathered people and says something. What does he say?

Spirituality for a Less Responsive Patient

If a person's mental or physical condition makes it seemingly impossible to communicate in words (possibly because of a coma or heavy sedation), there is a way to communicate spirituality that is referred to as "providing mutuality in the present." It means simply being with the person.

Just being with someone can have spiritual value because it conveys that the person is not alone, that there is hope because there is togetherness. This mutuality can communicate essential elements of spirituality by transforming the dread of abandonment and terror of isolation into hope. As Herbert Anderson has written, "It is the presence of this mutuality that is the secret of all our hopes and it is the absence of this mutuality that makes us hopeless."[12]

Words are not always necessary. Silence can be more valuable at times than words. Simply being present can be a very spiritual experience.

PRAYERS WITHOUT THEOLOGY

People in your care may occasionally ask you to pray for them. Caregivers need to be careful in responding so we don't impose our religious beliefs or deliver something that is quite different from what they ask or expect from us. One respectful response is to ask their permission to pray in your accustomed manner. You could say, "Would it be all right with you if I prayed in the way that is most familiar to me?"

Another way of responding could involve using prayers that do not use theological language. Some prayers can be worded in ways that are acceptable to people of any religious tradition. The body of these prayers has general language, but you could silently add an introduction and conclusion in the language of your religion or in any words that feel comfortable to you. Feel free to do that with the following prayers.

When someone in our care asks us to pray for her, she has a specific reason for making that request. She wants that prayer to be intended specifically for her, and she no doubt hopes the prayer will be effective. The following prayers, therefore, contain those three elements—they address a specific need, they have blanks where you would use the patient's name, and they acknowledge the prayer's effectiveness.

Prayer for Strength, Joy, and Comfort

I ask that in the midst of weakness, strength might be found. I pray that in the midst of sorrow, joy might be found. I pray that in the midst of pain, comfort might be found. Give _____ strength. Give _____ joy. Give _____ comfort. As I pray for _____, I sense the welling up of strength. I sense the welling up of joy. I sense the welling up of comfort. May this strength, joy, and comfort continue to build.

Prayer for Patience

I pray for patience. I ask for the granting of patience to _____. May his/her mind come to rest. May _____'s body find relaxation. May _____'s spirit know peace. May patience be _____'s assurance. We pray for that patience, giving thanks that that patience will in fact be a reality.

Prayer before an Operation

Strengthen _____ to do what he/she has to do and bear what he/she has to bear; that, accepting the skills and gifts of surgeons and nurses, _____ may be restored to usefulness in this world with a spirit of thanksgiving. Grant this acceptance. Grant this restoration. Grant this usefulness. Grant this thanksgiving. We pray in confidence that these requests will be granted.

Prayer for Relief from Pain

We offer a prayer for relief from pain. We ask that the pain which _____ feels might be lightened. Lift the pain. Soften the hard feelings. Ease the suffering. Bring comfort. Bring respite. Bring relief. As we pray, the pain is being soothed. Comfort is coming. Respite is coming. Relief is coming. _____ is feeling the comfort as it comes. _____ is feeling the relief as it comes. _____'s feelings are being lightened. His/her feelings are being softened. His/her feelings are being eased. A lightening. A softening. An easing. Comfort. Respite. Relief. It is happening as we pray.

Prayer for Sanctification

I pray that _____ may become fully aware of the presence of all holy powers. May those powers continue to grow in him/her. _____, you are being touched by the holy. _____, you are being held by the Divine. _____, you are being fully surrounded by all powers of sanctification. As I pray, this is all coming into being. Let it be now and always.

Prayer for the Granting of Release

Let us pray for release from this world. We pray that the family and friends of _____ might have the strength, the courage, the resolve to release _____ from their care. We pray that _____ might have the strength, the courage, the resolve to release him/herself from caring family and friends. We ask for trust. We ask for peace. All this we ask as we give thanks for the life of _____. In that thanksgiving and in love, we release _____. Grant him/her peace. Let it be.

CHAPTER NINE

The Right to Have a Sense of Family

In a time when "traditional" families have become less common, the standard definition of family needs to shift to reflect an accurate family portrait. Two-parent families with Dick, Jane, Sally, and Spot living behind the picket fence have become a vision of the past. Old questions of demographic composition and role identities are looking for new answers. Today we need a definition of family that is not limited by outdated demographics and rigid roles.

Any redefinition should emphasize connectedness, intimacy, and interdependence. A family need not be connected by blood, but some form of connectedness is important. A family today does not have to center around a sexual intimacy or a heterosexual intimacy, but some form of intimacy is important. A family need not be shaped by stereotypical roles of husband and wife and son and daughter, but some form of interdependence is very important. Whatever new definition "family" assumes, connectedness, intimacy, and interdependence will contribute vital meaning.

People in the last phases of life often do not enjoy a strong sense of connection, intimacy, or interdependence. They are frequently alone and isolated. They feel disconnected, unwanted, unneeded. But like all of us, they have a right to have a sense of family. As caregivers we need to help them enjoy this right.

The Lemon Sisters

Mildred, Margaret, and Betty were nicknamed "The Lemon Sisters" or, less kindly by a member of their nursing home staff, "The Sour Lemon Sisters." Other staff members and even some residents quickly adopted the nickname because the trio were such well-practiced complainers. They griped about meals, the nursing home's policies, and their "worthless" relatives who never visited. They shared gossip, sometimes quite malicious gossip, about individual staff members and residents.

Mildred, Margaret, and Betty were not sisters. They were not even related, but they were inseparably united through a commonality of shared complaints. In many ways, they formed a substitute family for the traditional families they felt they no longer had. Their connectedness was their common cause of complaining. They were intimate in sharing the most personal gossip about other people. They were interdependent in their encouragement of each other; each always found an audience in the other two.

When Margaret died, an irreplaceable member of the family was gone. Their little family would never be the same. Her special talent for snooping could not be replaced. Her biting witticisms would never be heard again. Her rapt attention as an audience for Mildred and Betty was lost for good. No one could be an adequate substitute for Margaret in their world. With her death, "The Lemon Sisters" were gone.

Rick

Family was always important to Rick. Growing up, he had been part of a tightly knit family. He tried to perpetuate that closeness with his three children, ages 14 through 18, by carrying on the family camping tradition that began when he was six, when his grandfather took him on his overnight trip to the woods.

"Heaven must be something like drinking a beer while sitting around the family campfire," Rick often said. He was convinced that he would once again be able to see his grandfather around some future campfire.

But Rick had been unable to camp for two years, and he faced the possibility that he would never be able to go camping with his family again. Soon after he had been admitted to a residential hospice facility, he made two requests that helped him communicate his heartfelt belief in family closeness. One involved his daily bath, the other involved campfires.

During the last week of his life, Rick's parents joined his wife and children from morning till night in his room. One morning a home health aide asked him if he was ready for his daily bath. Rick said he was ready, but he wanted his father to give him the bath.

Rick asked his father who, with a little embarrassment and a lot of love, agreed. His father had not given Rick a bath since he was a baby. Now, as he gently soaped and rinsed his grown son, Rick's father experienced his son's entire life passing before him.

A son's very loving request was met by an equally loving response from a father. Both request and response required *a great amount of emotional maturity, and both could only be fulfilled by people who knew connectedness, intimacy, and interdependence.*

Rick's other request was made two days before his death. He asked for a family campfire. The staff arranged for his bed to be moved to the hospice's living room and placed in front of the fireplace. Rick's 16-year-old son, who had been the most detached member of the family, helped in this most obviously physically painful move. Rick's brother brought a can of beer and gave Rick a straw so he could sip it. The family circled around Rick, his 16-year-old son held his father's hand, and Rick recalled some of the family's favorite campfire memories.

Rick's health deteriorated rapidly over the next two days. He moved in and out of consciousness, with occasional lucid moments. He died peacefully in his sleep. His family thought he was probably dreaming about their last campfire or perhaps some future family gathering around a campfire.

Doug

These are my own family stories.

My wife and I were determined to have the perfect child. We had waited more than three years, and we prepared for the birth of a child we knew would be the most intelligent, beautiful, well-behaved. Like many parents awaiting their first child, we read many books on child-rearing. My wife exercised and had a very healthy diet. We took Lamaze childbirth classes. We were even careful about the sounds in our environment and their possible contribution to the development of this child growing in the womb. We were certain that we would produce the perfect child.

Kristin was born about seven weeks prematurely and weighed just under six pounds. But these were only minor abnormalities compared with what we would soon learn about our daughter.

As soon as she was born, Kristin had an unusual cry—somewhat distant, eerie, high pitched. Her cry alerted the medical personnel that something more than prematurity was wrong. Within an hour after Kristin's birth, a nurse informed us that Kristin needed to be flown by helicopter—within the next 20 minutes—to a medical center some 50 miles away. We could be with Kristin for only the next 20 minutes.

We were in shock. We didn't know what to say to each other, what to do, what to imagine might explain this sudden development. The only thing we could think of doing was to have a baptism service in the hospital room. We baptized Kristin with our tears, and then we said good-bye to our daughter, our firstborn.

Over the next seven weeks, my wife and I spent many days driving those 50 miles to look at Kristin through a glass window. She was attached to several machines. We could only touch her if we wore masks and rubber gloves. From the outside, she looked tiny but fairly normal. But inside, her heart was deformed, she had four kidneys instead of the usual two, and her lungs were exceptionally small. Doctors also thought she had probable brain damage as well as many other physical problems.

Near the end of seven weeks, a pediatric cardiologist, Dr. Albers, told us that Kristin needed open-heart surgery within the week. Her size and various physical problems meant that she had only a 5 percent chance of surviving the surgery, but without the operation she could live not more than a couple of months. We had no choice but to give approval for the surgery.

Dr. Albers then surprised us with a beautiful gift. He said he wanted us to have Kristin with us the night before the operation. He wanted us to hold her because he felt that there was a wonderful healing power in touch. So we gratefully held Kristin for the entire night before her operation. We focused all our energy on sending our love to her. We gave her all the internal resources we had to give. Later we realized that Dr. Albers had intended that healing touch more for my wife and me than for Kristin.

The next morning arrived too soon. Three hours after Kristin was taken into the operating room, Dr. Albers emerged smiling. There was a bounce in his step. A miracle had occurred, he told us. Kristin made it through the operation and we would be able to see her soon.

But another hour passed. Then two hours. Dr. Albers at last came to us, but this time there was no smile, no bounce. Kristin's heart had stopped. They had to open her tiny chest again. She would be in our presence soon, he said, but his voice was full of foreboding.

Kristin was rolled past us toward her glass room. Her color was gray. A few minutes later, we sensed panic in her room. A voice announced, "Code blue." Suddenly everything was in motion. People rushed past us and surrounded Kristin. We saw blood on the hands and gowns of some people in her room. Then the commotion stopped. People slowly, silently, left her room one at a time until Dr. Albers was the only one left. After a few moments, he came to us with words that are forever locked in my mind: "We've lost her."

I gained a great deal from Kristin in those too-brief seven weeks. I expected her to be the most beautiful child. She taught me what beauty really is, and it has nothing to do with physical appearance or physical health. Although she was deformed, Kristin was indeed the most beautiful child I have ever seen.

I expected Kristin to be intelligent. Although she had serious brain damage, she taught me something about intelligence. From her, I learned more about myself and about life than I had ever learned from any college professor or scholarly book.

I also expected Kristin would be a well-behaved child. Through her, I learned that if a little child has life and health, good manners are just of minor importance. From Kristin, I learned a great deal about family—about connectedness, intimacy, and interdependence.

My second story

My dad was besieged with cancer, emphysema, heart problems, and steroid addiction. No one knew which would provide the final death blow, but everyone knew that it would arrive soon.

My father's macho manner is one of the many things I best remember about him. I could easily imagine a picture dictionary in which my dad's picture would illustrate the definition of "macho." He was a United States Naval Academy graduate who had fought in World War II and the Korean War. After Korea, he went to work for Caterpillar Tractors. He was always taller than I, always heavier, always stronger. His trademark facial expression came to be known as the "Bill Smith scowl."

Yet the times I remember and cherish most were those when his macho image melted. When I went to him in fear and trembling to ask his permission to go into the ministry, he unexpectedly told me that what I did was not as important as how I did it. He encouraged me to go into the ministry with all my heart and soul. He said that I would never disappoint him if I completely gave of myself in any pursuit.

After my baby daughter died, he came to me silently, with tears welling in his eyes. He stayed with me just long enough not to weep openly, but long enough for me to know that he was going to cry and needed to do it alone.

At my younger brother's funeral, our whole family was gathered at my parents' house. Dad asked me to go outside with him. He took me to the far end of the backyard. Looking me in the eyes, he told me how much he had loved my brother and how much he loved me. Then he threw his arms around me and shook in uncontrollable sobbing.

When my father's death approached, I decided to move back to where he lived. I moved into his house for a while to be close to him for the last nine months of his life. During that time together, we explored our connectedness, intimacy, and interdependence. We laughed together, cried, hugged, shared secrets, apologized, and forgave. We did not do all that we could have done, but we did much. We did enough.

His last days weren't pretty. He was extremely uncomfortable and looked terrible. He did not die peacefully. Yet he had done much with the life that was given him, and he had done much with the death that was given him.

My father died many years ago, but his presence stays with me. In my dreams, he always plays the role of advisor, guide, or judge. I am still seeking his advice, guidance, and approval. Apparently we still need our connectedness, intimacy, and interdependence. Family relationships do not end, even with death.

In our roles as caregivers—professional, friends, or family members—we need to promote connectedness, intimacy, and interdependence for those in our care, whatever form these "families" might take. In the following exercises and activities, the word family is used in the broadest possible sense; it includes not only blood relatives, but also friends, companions, caregivers—anyone who shares connectedness, intimacy, and interdependence with a person nearing the end of life.

Tools and techniques for promoting the right to have a sense of family

FAMILY STRENGTH ASSESSMENT

When we are around people for long periods of time, we tend to become more aware of their shortcomings. We notice the traits that others do not consciously want to reveal. This happens inevitably among families, especially when they must endure the added tensions of caring for someone who needs a lot of attention. In their interaction around caregiving tasks, family members can all too easily focus on each other's imperfections. Yet families can also rally during these difficult times and rise to an unexpectedly high level of functioning.

The following activity can help the family as a whole, or individual members, examine the positive qualities of the family and its members and discover ways to function most effectively. By exploring and emphasizing family strengths, we not only function better as a unit and as individual members, but we also come to appreciate our families more.

For the following family assessment, consider these five questions:

- What are the three greatest strengths of your family?
- How do members of your family complement one another, so that collectively you are stronger than you would be as individuals?
- What occasions from your family history have produced fond memories?
- How might various members of your community be envious of your family?
- If your family were to break apart, what would you miss the most?

SENTENCE COMPLETION

This activity can promote discussion of important issues within a family setting. Caregivers can encourage those in our care to complete the following sentences:

My (husband, wife, partner, companion, daughter, son, roommate) makes me happy when he/she

_____.

My _____ makes me sad when he/she

_____.

My _____ makes me angry when he/she

_____.

I would feel closer to my _____ if

_____.

My _____ would be more beneficial to me during this time if he/she _____.

Before I die, the one message I want to give to my _____ is _____.

Before I die, the one message I want to hear from my _____ is _____.

SHARING DREAMS

Several books about dreams and dying suggest that not only do people facing death often dream about death, but their family members also are likely to dream about it.

A useful exercise to increase the sense of family connectedness and intimacy involves setting a time once a week for families to gather and share their dreams. Each family member could describe one dream from the past week. Then all the other relatives could discuss their feelings and thoughts about that dream.

POSITIVE EXCHANGES

This activity requires two family members—one nearing the end of life and another relative—to help increase the number of positive exchanges between them. Each person would list five or six tasks that the other could do to please the one making the list. The tasks should be stated in positive terms rather than as complaints. Not all five or six tasks need to be completed, but the person who carries out the tasks should choose three that can be done within the coming week. You may want to do this activity every month.

FAMILY BACK MASSAGE

The entire family can participate in this activity, including the person in the last phases of life if it is feasible. Even if that person is unable to participate, the rest of the family can do it as a means of strengthening the bond of the family as a caregiving unit.

1. Gather everyone who feels the connectedness, intimacy, and interdependence and wants to participate.

2. One person lies facedown on a comfortable rug, with elbows out and hands near the head.

3. Everyone else kneels around him so that each person will massage a different area of his body.

4. The massagers take turns leading four minutes of massage as the others try to duplicate the leader's style. Make sure the entire body is massaged, including head, fingers, and toes. Everyone massages simultaneously, imitating the leader's style, using the same hand motions and pressure.

5. Take a 30-second pause between each leader's 4-minute session.

6. After each member of the family has had a turn at leading, let someone else receive the next massage.

7. After everyone has had a turn to be massaged, some verbal sharing may take place, or everyone can start doing massages all over again.

GIFT GIVING

This activity can tell much about a family as it helps to strengthen the family unit.

A caregiver would suggest that each family member think of one to three gifts that he can give to the entire family. It should be a joy to give as well as to receive, not a gift that the giver thinks they "ought" to want. The gift can be an object, such as a book, an artwork, a video, a meal; or it can be an action, such as doing a chore, giving hugs to everyone, writing a poem, singing a song for the family.

After each person has received a gift, he verbally expresses appreciation. When all the gifts have been given and received, the caregiver can initiate and guide a discussion about the process.

THE IDEAL FAMILY

As caregiver, you could present the following suggestions to someone in your care.

> There is an assignment that I am inviting you to do. Over the next week, I would like you to write a description of your family when it is functioning at its best level. Describe something that you feel is possible to achieve but is not being achieved presently. Describe each member of your family operating at his or her best. Describe how each person would interact with every other family member. Go into lots of detail. Let your imagination take over and run freely as you portray your

ideal family, an ideal that you feel is possible to achieve. The next time we are together, we will spend some time reviewing and talking about your description.

The description generated by this activity can be used as a basis for the family's plan of care. It can be used like a blueprint that will bring the family closer to the person's ideal description. If the whole family does not want to take part in this comprehensive plan of care, individual family members can incorporate the parts that pertain to them.

FAMILY MEMBER ROLE DEFINITION

When a relative or loved one nears the end of life, other family members often become confused about what their roles should be at this time. "What does my (wife, parent, brother) want me to do? What is my caregiving role?" we may ask ourselves. The relative who needs our care may be just as confused. Often both of us feel awkward in just asking these new, unfamiliar questions.

This activity can help clarify our roles. Of the two forms that follow, the caregiver should first decide which one is more appropriate for the person being cared for, then give it to her and ask her to fill it out and return it.

Family Helper Role Definition

From the following list of items that you, the care recipient, might receive from _____ in your family, put an "x" beside those that best complete this statement: "I would like _____ to help me. . . ." Cross out any item that you feel you will never want from this caregiver. Put a question mark next to any you are unsure about. Use the blank space for anything else you wish to say.

I would like _____ to help me. . .

_____ do some handyman projects;

_____ finish a project (_____);

_____ purchase food and prepare meals;

_____ exercise some of my muscles;

_____ maintain a clean, safe environment;

_____ do some errands outside my home;

_____ take on some little outings;

_____ with my personal grooming;

_____ by reading to me;

_____ write some letters;

_____ discuss _____ with me;

_____ by touching and holding me often;

_____ by _____.

Family Partner Role Definition

From the following list of items that you, the care recipient, might receive from your partner, put an "x" beside those that best complete this statement: "I would like my partner to help me. . . ." Cross out any item that you feel you will never want from your partner. Put a question mark next to any you are unsure about. Use the blank space for anything else you wish to say:

I would like my partner to help me. . .

_____ do some handyman projects;

_____ finish a project (_____);

_____ purchase food and prepare meals;

_____ exercise some of my muscles;

_____ maintain a clean, safe environment;

_____ do some errands outside my home;

_____ take some little outings;

_____ with my personal grooming;

_____ by occasionally reading to me;

_____ write some letters;

_____ to discuss _____ with me;

_____ by touching and holding me often;

_____ remember our times of intimacy;

_____ give and receive sexual satisfaction;

_____ by _____.

The Family Life Review

This activity uses the technique of bringing the past into the present as a means of enhancing a current sense of family. Suggest the following to the person in your care:

- Describe what you consider to be your best family vacation as a child.

- Describe the best holiday you ever spent with your family as a child.

- Describe your most memorable positive experience with your father.
- Describe your most memorable positive experience with your mother.
- How would you define what you consider to be your "family" right now?
- When were you most aware of a strong degree of interdependence within your present family? Elaborate.
- When were you most aware of a strong degree of intimacy within your present family? Elaborate.
- What time or event are you excitedly anticipating that will be spent with your present family?

COUPONS

Family members could present a person in the last phase of life with three coupons, redeemable whenever the recipient chooses. Here are some samples, but you are encouraged to invent your own.

- "This coupon is good for a 10-minute back massage."
- "This coupon is good for one ice-cream cone. You choose the flavor."
- "This coupon entitles you to have me as your slave for a whole afternoon."
- "This coupon means that I will read to you for an hour from a book of your choice."
- "This coupon is good for a manicure."

- "This coupon means that I will be the guardian of your peace and quiet for a whole day."
- "This coupon entitles you to a three-hour outing to a location of your choice."

THE FIVE-CARD ACTIVITY

This exercise can help family members understand the dying process from the point of view of the person who is facing death. It helps the rest of the family realize how a dying person experiences the gradual letting go of all that is important and valuable.

Family members can do this activity together, but each participant does the first four steps individually. A family discussion is the fifth step.

1. Write down the five most precious things in your life. These might be possessions like a home or a job; they might be certain people; or they could be states of being or qualities, such as intelligence, a sense of humor, or health. Write each item on a separate sheet of paper, which should remain confidential.

2. Then ponder the meaning of each of the five most precious items and decide which is the least important. Discard the paper on which that item is written by placing it face down in front of you. Close your eyes and try to imagine what life would be like without this person, thing, or quality.

3. Now consider the values of the remaining four items in the same way. Decide which is the least important, discard that paper, and try to imagine life without it.

4. Repeat the same process with the remaining three items.

5. After discarding the third item, family members could discuss with each other some of the feelings you had in deciding what to discard and how you felt about life without these things. Then the discussion should move into the area of imagining what similar feelings the dying person is having.

This activity portrays quite accurately what many dying people experience. They know they lack time, health, and energy, and they must make difficult decisions that are forced on them. Tough choices must be made soon. There is never enough time, health, or energy to enjoy everything they want to enjoy or to see everyone they wish to see. It is important that caregivers and loved ones understand how the gradual disillusionment of dying can be most difficult.

I Can Be My Own Family

A caregiver can assign "homework" of completing eight sentences, each beginning, "I need my family to _____." For example: "I need my family to show me more patience. I need my family to prepare my meals for me. I need my family to give me more opportunities to laugh."

From the list of eight, three needs should be selected as things that the person in your care can make into personal goals. Each statement would be reworded to reflect goals that she can achieve herself. For example: "I need to show myself more patience. I need to prepare my own meals for myself. I need to give myself more opportunities to laugh."

After the new statements are composed, she would map out a strategy for accomplishing those objectives herself. Or, several strategies might be incorporated to move toward reaching those goals.

FAMILY DISCUSSION

This activity begins with family members gathering pencil and paper and writing at the top of a page, "My Opinions Concerning Death." Each person then writes for 15 to 20 minutes. Suggest that they follow a stream-of-consciousness style—they should not worry about sentence structure, spelling, or punctuation, just scribble the thoughts down on paper as they come to mind. If anyone has difficulty getting started, the following questions may help generate some ideas.

- What causes people to die?
- What is the worst death that you can imagine?
- What is the best death that you can imagine?
- What is your opinion about an afterlife?

When everyone has finished writing, each person shares what he or she has written with the rest of the family. No value judgments or critical comments are allowed. Everyone's opinion is accepted as having equal value and validity with everyone else's.

LETTING GO AT THE TIME OF DEATH

Most of us hold in our tears. We don't want to let go of our internal grip on emotional control, and we don't want to give up our external attachment to the people we love. Often when death comes very near, we think we are exercising internal self-control for the sake of someone else—a relative, friend, or our dying loved one. As caregivers we might provide family members or other caregivers the following litany to help relieve some of the pressure that builds with the difficult process of letting go.

When death is near, a spokesperson from the family or care team is selected to lead this litany, beginning each sentence with the name of the dying person.

Spokesperson: _____,
   in knowing that you have led a good and
   complete life,
Family: We release you.
Spokesperson: _____,
   in knowing that we care for your total
   well-being,
Family: We release you.
Spokesperson: _____,
   in knowing that we are doing what is best
   for you,
Family: We release you.
Spokesperson: _____,
   in knowing that we are not at all angry
   with you,
Family: We release you.
Spokesperson: _____,
   in knowing that you have all our love,
Family: We release you.

continued

> *Spokesperson:* _____,
>   *in knowing that there is no more that we can do*
>   *for you,*
> *Family:* We release you.
> *Spokesperson:* _____,
>   *in knowing that your pain will soon be relieved,*
> *Family:* We release you.

This exercise can be important for future reference for a family or care team. Keeping a copy of this litany can help mourners later if they feel guilty or have some unresolved feelings. Reviewing this litany can have ongoing psychological benefits: They will realize that potential issues of unfinished business were addressed. Love was expressed. The time was right. We did it together.

From Mourning to Disengaging

When death finally does occur, the family experience intense mourning as a result of their loss. The following guided imagery activity can be led by a caregiver to help family members relieve some of the intensity of their grieving.

> ### The Entrustment
> Close your eyes and center your concentration on your breathing. . . . Feel the coolness and freshness of each breath that you inhale into your lungs. . . . Feel the warmth

and heaviness of each breath that you exhale. . . . Feel the freshness coming in and the heaviness going out. . . .

In a little while I am going to lead you through an imaginary experience. You will be imagining some people. Besides picturing yourself in this experience, you will also picture someone who has died recently, someone you have loved very much. You will also be picturing another person, someone different from the person who has died. This other person will be the most loving person you can imagine, the most loving person who can come into your imagination. So there will be three central people in this imagery experience: yourself, someone who has recently died, and the most loving person you can possibly imagine. . . .

Now picture in your mind the most loving person you can possibly imagine. Picture this loving person standing in front of you. . . . Imagine this loving person standing before you with arms stretching toward you.

Now imagine that there are hundreds of people standing in a line behind this loving person. The line of people extends far into the distance and disappears into a bright, warm, yellow light. You see this long line of hundreds of people disappearing into a bright, warm, yellow light. . . .

In your arms you are holding someone who has died, someone to whom you have felt very close. The body is very light in weight. . . . You are looking at this person in your arms, this person who has died, this person
continued

to whom you have felt very close. . . . You are reminded of some special moments that you shared with this person. Picture in your mind a few of those special times. . . . Look once again at this person in your arms. In your imagination, say good-bye to this person as you say the person's name. Say good-bye to this person to whom you have felt very close.

You now carry this body over to the loving person with outstretched arms. You gently place the dead body in the outstretched arms and watch the body being passed along the line of people toward that bright, warm, yellow light. The body is gently and carefully passed from one person to another. . . . The body is now passed into the light. You see the light become brighter and warmer as the body enters the light. You know that the body is now safe, very safe. . . .

You look once again at the loving person across from you. That person shares a warm and accepting smile and says, "Thank you. Your friend is very safe. So it is okay for you to go now." You turn around and begin walking away from this place. As you are leaving, you once again become aware of your breathing. . . .

Feel the coolness and freshness of each breath that you inhale into your lungs. . . . Feel the warmth and heaviness of each breath that you exhale from your lungs. . . . Feel the freshness come in and the heaviness go out. . . . After feeling the cleansing quality of your breathing for a little while longer, you may slowly open your eyes. . . .

FROM DISENGAGING TO REVITALIZING

Here is another imagery experience that caregivers could use to help diminish the intensity of the mourning process.

THE FUNERAL SERVICE

Close your eyes and concentrate on your breathing. . . . Feel the coolness and freshness of each breath that you inhale into your lungs. . . . Feel the warmth and heaviness of each breath that you exhale. . . . Feel the freshness coming in and the heaviness going out. . . .

In your imagination, you are standing with a group of friends and relatives in a cemetery. You look around and see many of your friends and relatives. . . . This is a funeral service, a funeral service for someone who has recently died, someone with whom you have been very close. . . . Whose funeral is this? . . . How do you feel being at this person's funeral?

The funeral service is ending. People are leaving. Yet you decide that you want to stay for a while at the graveside. . . . You look at the freshly turned earth from the grave, and you see all the trees and green grass all around you. . . . There are many trees in this cemetery. One particular tree on a small hill catches your attention. You walk over and sit underneath this tree and look out across this green cemetery. . . . You are resting, and you feel very peaceful in this place. You are breathing in some very peaceful air. . . .

continued

After a short while, a chipmunk comes up in front of you and looks at you rather curiously while it nibbles an acorn. . . . You think that the chipmunk is funny looking and you imagine that the chipmunk thinks you look rather funny, too. . . . In your imagination, you now become that chipmunk nibbling on that acorn. You are the chipmunk nibbling on the acorn. . . .

As a chipmunk, you start running through the grass . . . . Up ahead, you see another chipmunk and decide, mischievously, to chase it up a nearby tree. The two of you go around and around and around the tree trunk until you reach a topmost branch. You can no longer see the other chipmunk. Yet at the end of that high branch, you see a bright red cardinal. The cardinal turns its head toward you and looks at you rather curiously. You think the cardinal looks rather funny, and you imagine that the cardinal thinks you look funny, too . . . . In your imagination, you now become that cardinal perched at the end of that branch. . . .

As a cardinal, you flap your wings and leap off the branch into the air. You test your wings and soar and dive, soar and dive. You fly to the right, you fly to the left, up and down, up and down again. As you are flying, look at everything that you are flying over. . . . Feel the warmth of the sun. . . . See the beautiful blue sky. . . . Smell the freshness of the air. . . .

As you are smelling the freshness of the air, feel that freshness and coolness as you inhale into your lungs. . . .

> Feel the warmth and heaviness of each breath that you exhale. . . . Feel the freshness come in and the heaviness go out and, when you are ready to return to this room in the fresh, living present, you may slowly open your eyes. . . .

THE LAMINATED ANGEL

As a caregiver, you undoubtedly are not the only one dispensing care and attention. But you may feel alone from time to time. Caregivers often need to alert the rest of the caregiving team of their own individual needs. One way to do that is by having each member of the team cut out a piece of cardboard in the shape of an angel (or, for the less artistically inclined, cut a picture of an angel out of a magazine, catalogue, or greeting card) and laminate it. When a caregiver needs special attention—for whatever reason—the laminated angel is pinned onto the clothing. The laminated angel signals other caregivers to approach this particular caregiver gently, say kind words, give hugs, and help in whatever way possible. This is an easy yet generous way to ease the caregiver's load on that particular day.

Chapter Ten

Conclusion

Dean

I did not know my brother Dean too well when we were kids because I was the oldest of five boys and he was the youngest. Because of our 14-year difference in age, I was determined to know him better as an adult.

In 1980, Dean was a student at the University of Wisconsin, and I lived and worked in Phoenix, Arizona. I decided early that autumn that I wanted him to visit me during his Christmas vacation. I would pay for his round-trip ticket, and we could go bicycling in the desert. I thought he'd like that. But one thing or another got in my way. I was busy at work, and I never got around to inviting him. Christmas came and went. An opportunity too quickly lost.

Late the next summer, I decided once again that I ought to invite Dean to visit during his Christmas break. This time I fantasized about the particular areas of the desert that might be best for bicycling. I even planned possible routes. Once again, I got sidetracked and never got around to picking up the phone and inviting him. Another opportunity had slipped away.

In January 1982, I actually wrote an entry on my calendar for September 1: "Call Dean." This time I would definitely nail down arrangements for bringing him to Phoenix.

On July 30, 1982, Dean died in a fire. I would never see my youngest brother again. I would never have a chance to know him any better. He and I would never cycle through the desert. Opportunities had been there, and then they suddenly disappeared in tragedy.

Throughout this book we have examined opportunities for assuring the rights of people nearing death. I never had the opportunity to know Dean as well as I had wanted. And I certainly never had a chance to know or help him at the sudden end of his life. That is perhaps why I feel so strongly about making the most of any opportunity that caregivers can seize to help people in the last phases of life.

Caregivers may never know the extent of the benefits they extend to their loved ones and patients when we allow them their final rights and give them opportunities to exercise those rights. But not knowing doesn't mean we shouldn't try. Opportunities to facilitate those rights are with us now, but they soon may be gone.

To inspire us to put into practice what we have learned from these pages, I would like to review some key points briefly. First we examined the right to be in control. We saw how Martha, Phyllis, Charlie, and Cathy wanted and used this right in different ways. Martha wanted the right to control how she was perceived and what was said in her presence. Phyllis wanted to control her emotional responses to her coming death. Charlie wanted to control how his pain was to be relieved. Cathy wanted to control how she fought a battle that everyone else had stopped waging.

They deserved, as much as any of us, to have their right to be in control honored. They deserved not to have caregivers impose their ways of thinking, their behavior, or their will. As caregivers we have wonderful opportunities to allow and respect our patients' and loved ones' rights to be in control. These opportunities are with us now, but may not be much longer.

We looked at a person's right to have a sense of purpose. We saw that people in the final phases of life often have lost jobs, family roles, and abilities. We discussed their very real, immediate need for a sense of purpose to balance or replace those losses. Several ways were suggested, such as recalling the past and bringing former pleasant feelings into the present, that can create a sense of purpose in the current situation, even if the person has depleted strength or energy. These alternative ways allow a dying person opportunities to feel like a living person, one who can have positive effects on others. These opportunities are with us now, but may not be much longer.

We considered the right to know the truth. We met Glenda and Vicky who, like most of us, wanted to know what was happening to them and what would most likely happen to them in the near future. We recognized that people nearing the end of life experience many uncertainties and unknowns. Yet they need to know whatever can be known. They have a right to know about their own reality. We saw how an open sharing of the truth can promote cooperation between the person receiving care, family members, and caregivers. Together they can become equal partners in this venture.

Another essential final right is the right to comfort. We considered a wide variety of choices that people can make in searching for ways to find comfort. For Russell, it was oatmeal and butter. For Andy, acupuncture. For Elmer, reflexology. For Donald, an unshakable faith in God. We discovered how important it is for caregivers to offer as many choices as possible for finding comfort. We can even help create choices where people might think they have none, especially by offering choices in managing their own physical and emotional well-being. We also saw how we need to be open to accepting and honoring any coping style to help a person secure the right to be comfortable.

We also explored the right to touch and be touched. We acknowledged that we tend to have a misconception about when touch is most needed. We often fail to realize that this need both increases with age and is accentuated during times of stress and isolation. The desire for touch often seems overwhelming for many people nearing the end of life. For others, we recognize, the need for touch may be less strong. But enough people have this desire that we should recognize that right and give them as many opportunities to touch and be touched as they wish. These opportunities are available now, but may not be much longer.

People nearing the end of life don't lose their enjoyment of humor. As we laughed with Harry, we found, in fact, that the right to laughter is important to the sick and dying. We deprive them of that right if we constantly hide behind a mask of seriousness. We rob them of some of their humanity, we exclude them from the valuable ordinariness of being human, if we banish laughter from their lives. Like touch, humor is not desired all the time or by every individual. But we can use humor effectively if we are careful about its appropriateness. If we sense that our patients and loved ones want laughter, we should provide such opportunities.

In discussing the right to cry and express anger, we discovered that many people nearing death are not allowed the time or place to express the deep sadness and anger that they are experiencing. Caregivers need to allow and respect their right to express these emotions, and we should present them with opportunities to do so.

The right to explore spirituality is usually recognized by families and caregivers as our loved ones and patients approach death, but too often we unintentionally impose our own beliefs. This can stifle their own spiritual expression and growth. As caregivers, we should respect their right to explore and express their unique spirituality in any way they wish. We should look on spirituality through the broadest possible lens so that we can give our patients and loved ones opportunities for its fullest expression. We saw how broad spirituality can be through the experiences of Hazel and her watchful eyes, through Jack and his mystifying magic, through Jim and his ecclesiastically astute neighborhood barroom, and through David and his voracious appetite for religion. In allowing people nearing death the right to be spiritual and have their spiritual style respected, we caregivers also give ourselves opportunities for our own growth.

Last, we examined the right to have a sense of family. We saw how essential it is for everyone to feel connectedness, intimacy, and interdependence. This right was not placed last on the list unintentionally. It ties the other eight rights together, in fact, and helps assure them. In carrying out our daily caregiving work, we participate in connectedness, intimacy, and interdependence with those in our care. These essential ingredients comprise one's sense of family. If we caregivers share in that sense of family we will naturally feel compelled to offer and ensure the other final rights: the right to be in control, to have a sense of purpose, to know the truth, to be comfortable, to touch and be touched, to laugh, to cry and express anger, to be spiritual, and to have a sense of family. Within the human family, some of us are caregivers and others receive our care.

For those of us who are caregivers by choice or by fate, many opportunities lie before us. They are with us now, but they may not be here much longer. Let us take advantage of opportunities to share with people who mean so much to us. Let us take advantage of opportunities to share in the final phase of someone's life.

Let us take their final rights and turn them into opportunities— opportunities to exercise control, to find a sense of purpose, to explore the truth, to be comfortable, to touch and be touched, to laugh, to express emotions, to grow spiritually, and to enjoy connectedness, intimacy, and interdependence.

NOTES

1. Anne Wilson Schaef, *Beyond Therapy, Beyond Science.* (New York: HarperCollins, 1992).

2. Avery Weisman, *The Coping Capacity.* (New York: Human Sciences Press, 1984).

3. Adapted from John O. Stevens, *Awareness: Exploring, Experimenting, Experiencing.* (Moab, Utah: Real People Press, 1971).

4. Fritz Perls, *Gestalt Therapy Verbatim.* (Moab, Utah: Real People Press, 1969).

5. *The Complete Works of Chaung Tzu*, trans. B. Watson. (New York: Columbia University Press, 1968).

6. Adapted from L. M. Moleski, "Imagery Techniques in the Windsong Teachings," in *Anthology of Imagery Techniques,* ed. A. A. Sheikh. (Milwaukee: American Imagery Institute, 1986).

7. Philip Kapleau, *The Wheel of Life and Death.* (New York: Doubleday, 1989).

8. Doug Smith and Michael F. Maher, "Achieving a Healthy Death: The Dying Person's Attitudinal Contributions." (*The Hospice Journal* [1993] 9[1]: 21–32).

9. Kaye Herth, "Contributions of Humor As Perceived by the Terminally Ill." (*The American Journal of Hospice Care* [1990] 7[1]: 36–40).

10. Judith Lief, "Attentive Care: Working with the Dying Patient." (*Naropa Institute Journal of Psychology* [1985] 3: 11–17).

11. Donald Curtis, *The Christ-Based Teachings.* (Unity Village, Miss.: Unity Books, 1976).

12. Herbert Anderson, "After the Diagnosis: An Operational Theology for the Terminally Ill." (*Journal of Pastoral Care* [1989] 40[2]: 141–150).

RESOURCES

The following resources may be helpful to caregivers and families who want to explore more of the literature about death and dying.

Andersen, H., and P. MacElveen-Hoehn. (1988). "Gay clients with AIDS: New challenges for hospice programs." *The Hospice Journal* 4(2): 37–54.

Anderson, H. (1989). "After the diagnosis: An operational theology for the terminally ill." *Journal of Pastoral Care* 40(2): 141–150.

Boerstler, R. W., and H. S. Kornfeld. (1995). *Life to Death*. Rochester, VT: Healing Arts Press.

Burns, S. (1991). "The spirituality of dying." *Health Progress* 5: 48–54.

Byock, I. (1997). *Dying Well*. New York: Riverhead Books.

Callahan, M., and P. Kelly. (1992). *Final Gifts*. New York: Bantam Books.

Cassidy, S. (1991). *Sharing the Darkness*. New York: Orbis Books.

Cousins, N. (1979). *Anatomy of an Illness*. New York: W. W. Norton.

Duda, D. (1987). *Coming Home: A Guide to Dying at Home with Dignity*. New York: Aurora Press.

Fakouri, C., and P. Jones. (1987). "Relaxation Rx: Slow stroke back rub." *Journal of Gerontological Nursing* 19: 32–35.

Feinstein, D., and P. E. Mayo. (1990). *Rituals for Living and Dying*. San Francisco: HarperCollins.

Gonda, T. A., and J. E. Ruark. (1984). *Dying Dignified*. New York: Addison-Wesley.

Herth, K. (1990). "Contributions of humor as perceived by the terminally ill." *The American Journal of Hospice Care* 7(1): 36–40.

Hinton, J. M. (1963). "The physical and mental distress of the dying." *Quarterly Journal of Medicine* 32: 1–21.

Johanne de Montigny (1993). "Distress, stress and solidarity in palliative care." *Omega: Journal of Death and Dying* 27(1): 5–15.

Kalish, R. A. (1981). *Death, Grief, and Caring Relationships*. Monterey, Calif.: Brooks/Cole.

Kapleau, P. (1989). *The Wheel of Life and Death*. New York: Doubleday.

Kessler, D. (1997). *The Rights of the Dying*. New York: Macmillan.

Kramer, K. P. (1988). *The Sacred Art of Dying*. New York: Paulist Press.

Kramer, K. P. (1993). *Death Dreams*. New York: Paulist Press.

Kubler-Ross, E. (1971) *On Death and Dying*. New York: Macmillan.

Levine, S. (1982). *Who Dies?* New York: Anchor Books.

Leviton, D. (1986). "Thanatological theory and my dying father." *Omega: Journal of Death and Dying* 17(2): 127–144.

Lief, J. (1985). "Attentive care: Working with the dying patient." *Naropa Institute Journal of Psychology* 3: 11–17.

Longaker, C. (1997). *Facing Death and Finding Hope.* New York: Doubleday.

Magno, J. B. (1990). "The hospice concept of care: Facing the 1990s." *Death Studies* 14(2): 109–119.

Maher, M. F., and D. Smith. (1993). "I could have died laughing." *Journal of Humanistic Education and Development* 31: 123–129.

Maher, M. F., and D. C. Smith. (1994). "Psycho-palliating and anger." *Illness, Crisis and Loss* 4: 38–44.

Mauritzen, J. (1988). "Pastoral care for the dying and bereaved." *Death Studies* 12(2): 111–122.

Moore, T. (1992). *Care of the Soul.* New York: HarperCollins.

Mudd, P. (1990). "The dark self: Death as a transferential factor." *Journal of Analytical Psychology* 35: 125–141.

Nabe, C. (1989). "Health care and the transcendent." *Death Studies* 13: 557–565.

Nouwen, H. J. M. (1972). *The Wounded Healer.* Garden City, N.Y.: Doubleday.

Nuland, S. B. (1994). *How We Die.* New York: Alfred A. Knopf.

O'Brien, M. E. (1993). "Don't do everything possible for me." *The American Journal of Hospice and Palliative Care* 10(3): 8.

O'Connor, P. (1993). "A clinical paradigm for exploring spiritual concerns." In *Death and Spirituality*, edited by A. A. Sheikh, 133–141. Amityville, N.Y.: Baywood Publishing.

Older, J. (1982). *Touching Is Healing*. New York: Stein and Day.

Propst, L. R. (1980). "The comparative efficacy of religious and nonreligious imagery for the treatment of mild depression in religious individuals." *Cognitive Therapy and Research* 4: 167–178.

Rando, T. A. (1984). *Grief, Dying, and Death*. Champaign, Ill.: Research Press.

Reisz, H. F., Jr. (1992). "A dying person is a living person: A pastoral theology for ministry to the dying." *The Journal of Pastoral Care* 46(2): 184–192.

Robinson, V. M. (1986). "Humor is a serious business." *Dimensions of Critical Care Nursing* 5(3): 132–133.

Rosenthal, T. (1974). *How Could I Not Be Among You?* New York: George Braziller.

Saunders, C. M. (1978). "Terminal care." In *Psychosocial Care of the Dying Patient*, edited by C. A. Garfield, 22–33. New York: McGraw-Hill.

Seravalli, E. P. (1988). "The dying patient, the physician, and the fear of death." *New England Journal of Medicine* 319(26): 1728–1730.

Schaef, A. W. (1992). *Beyond Therapy, Beyond Science*. New York: HarperCollins.

Shneidman, E. S. (1977). "Aspects of the dying process." *Psychiatric Annals* 7(8): 391–397.

Smith, D. C. (1993a). "Exploring the religious-spiritual needs of the dying." *Counseling and Values* 37(2): 71–77.

Smith, D. C. (1993b). "The power of touch." *Caring Magazine* 12(11): 62.

Smith, D. C. (1993c). "The terminally ill patient's right to be in denial." *Omega: Journal of Death and Dying* 27(2): 115–121.

Smith, D. C. (1994a). "A 'last rights' group for persons with AIDS." *Journal for Specialists in Group Work* 19: 17–21.

Smith, D. C. (1994b). "Pain control and personal control." *Illness, Crisis and Loss* 4: 69–76.

Smith, D. C. (1994c). *The Tao of Dying*. Washington, D.C.: Caring Publications.

Smith, D. C., and L. A. Frisbie. (1994d). "The use of hypnosis with the terminally ill." *Medical Hypnoanalysis Journal* 9: 12–18.

Smith, D. C., and M. F. Maher. (1991a). "Group process and techniques with caregivers of the dying: The 'phoenix' alternative." *Journal for Specialists in Group Work* 16(3): 191–196.

Smith, D. C., and M. F. Maher. (1991b). "Healthy death." *Counseling and Values* 36(1): 42–48.

Smith, D. C., and M. F. Maher. (1993a). "Achieving a healthy death: The dying person's attitudinal contributions." *The Hospice Journal* 9(1): 21–32.

Smith, D. C., and M. F. Maher. (1993b). "On terminal illness and the patient's right to maintain control." *Illness, Crisis and Loss* 2(4): 47–51.

Smith, D. C., W. Richards, and M. F. Maher. (1993). "Metaphoric language: Palliation for the terminally ill." *Illness, Crisis and Loss* 2(4): 38–44.

Sogyal Rinpoche. (1992). *The Tibetan Book of Living and Dying.* New York: HarperCollins.

Thorson, J. A. (1985). "A funny thing happened on the way to the morgue: Some thoughts on humor and death, and a taxonomy of the humor associated with death." *Death Studies* 9: 201–216.

Vailiant, G. (1977). *Adaptation to Life.* Boston: Little, Brown.

Von Franz, M. (1987). *On Dreams and Death.* Translated by E. X. Kennedy. Boston: Shambhala.

Wasow, M. (1984). "Get out of my potato patch: A biased view of death and dying." *Health and Social Work* 9(4): 261–267.

Weenolsen, P. (1996). *The Art of Dying.* New York: St. Martin's Press.

Weisberg, J., and M. R. Haberman. (1989). "A therapeutic hugging week in a geriatric facility." *Journal of Gerontological Social Work* 13: 181–186.

Weisman, A. D. (1972). *On Dying and Denying.* New York: Behavioral Publications.

Weisman, A. D. (1984). *The Coping Capacity.* New York: Human Sciences Press.

Wholihan, D. (1992). "The value of reminiscence in hospice care." *The American Journal of Hospice and Palliative Care* 9(2): 33–35.

INDEX